PRAISE FOR
O. J. BRIGANCE

"[O. J. Brigance's] courageous fight against ALS is an inspiration to Americans all across the country."

—President Barack Obama at a White House reception for the Baltimore Ravens

"O. J. Brigance is my greatest inspiration. He is my hero. He proved that in football, and in life, you can do anything if you believe it can be done. His strength, his outlook, and his remarkable faith serve as examples of everything we should strive for in our own lives." —Ray Lewis, from the Foreword

"I am honored to call O. J. Brigance a friend and teammate. Everyone in the Ravens organization knows that O. J. Brigance is the strongest man in the building, and it's a building of a lot of strong men. O.J. remains incredibly strong both spiritually and intellectually. I am energized by his presence and what he brings to the team and to my life. O.J. is our greatest motivation and our greatest inspiration, and we are all blessed to be able to share in his light." —Coach John Harbaugh, Baltimore Ravens

STRENGTH

OF A

CHAMPION

FINDING FAITH AND FORTITUDE
THROUGH ADVERSITY

O. J. BRIGANCE

with PETER SCHRAGER

 New American Library

New American Library
Published by the Penguin Group
Penguin Group (USA) LLC, 375 Hudson Street,
New York, New York 10014

USA | Canada | UK | Ireland | Australia | New Zealand | India | South Africa | China
penguin.com
A Penguin Random House Company

Published by New American Library, a division of Penguin Group (USA) LLC.
Previously published in a New American Library hardcover edition.

First New American Library Trade Paperback Printing, October 2014

All photos courtesy of the Brigance Brigade Foundation except as follows: Raymond Ebai: p. 7 middle right, bottom, p. 8 top; Phil Hoffman: p. 3 middle, bottom left, bottom right, p. 4 top, p. 7 top right, middle left; Jim McCue/Maryland Jockey Club: p. 4 middle; Paul Morris: page 1 bottom; Sarah Gubara/Maroon PR: p. 5 top, middle left, bottom; Eve Hemsley/Maroon PR: p. 5 middle right, p. 6 top; Sharon Redmond/photographybysharon.com: p. 6 middle; Marlene Alvarez/Maroon PR: p. 6 bottom; Shawn Hubbard/Baltimore Ravens: p. 4 bottom, p. 8 middle left; Official White House photo by Pete Souza: page 8 bottom

THE LIBRARY OF CONGRESS HAS CATALOGUED THE HARDCOVER EDITION AS FOLLOWS:
Brigance, O. J., 1969–
Strength of a champion: finding faith and fortitude through adversity/
O. J. Brigance, Peter Schrager; [foreword by] Ray Lewis.
p. cm.
ISBN 978-0-451-46761-4 (hardback)
1. Brigance, O. J., 1969– 2. Football players—United States—Biography.
3. Amyotrophic lateral sclerosis—Patients—Biography. 4. Football players—
Religious life—United States. I. Schrager, Peter. II. Title.
GV939.B728A3 2013
796.332092—dc23   2013025873
[B]

Set in Janson Text
Designed by Spring Hoteling

For the God Most High and the Queen B.

FOREWORD

BY RAY LEWIS

I'VE been blessed to have many opportunities in my life, but there's been no single honor as humbling as being asked to write the foreword to O. J. Brigance's book.

O.J. is my greatest inspiration. He is my hero. He is the embodiment of the complete man.

We first met in the summer of 2000, when O.J. signed as a free agent with the Ravens. We hit it off in the linebackers room and immediately connected. As we got closer, I called him "Juice" and he called me "Sugar." We went on to hoist the Lombardi Trophy together as teammates and brothers. Juice wasn't the biggest or fastest guy on the team, but no person on the football field was ever smarter or worked harder than him. He proved that in football, and in life, you can do anything if you believe it can be done. He was the consummate teammate—reliable, trustworthy, forever by your side.

When O.J. was first diagnosed with ALS in 2007, he asked me not to treat him any differently than how I'd treated him beforehand. I never have. We still joke around all the time, and though he can no longer use his voice, we continue to communicate on a daily basis. Whether it's through an e-mail he sends me to start my day, a message he shares through his machine, or the presence of his unmistakable smile, O.J. speaks to me. ALS has robbed him of the use of his extremities and the ability to talk like you or me, but it hasn't stopped him from living his life to the fullest.

What O.J. might not know is just how important he is to me and the Baltimore Ravens organization as a whole. He's our guiding light, a beautiful positive force that motivates us to be better players and to be better men. His courage is invigorating. His positivity is contagious. O. J. Brigance was more than merely a piece to the 2013 Baltimore Ravens Super Bowl championship puzzle. He was our heart and soul. Ask any individual within the Ravens organization who their role model is, and they'll all respond with one name and one name only: *Juice.*

As a man, O.J. is everything I aspire to be. This man motivates me to be the very best—at whatever I'm doing—every single day. His strength, his outlook, and his remarkable faith serve as examples of everything we should strive for in our own lives.

He inspires me to never complain. To never worry. To never gossip. To never waver. To never lose faith. I can't tell you where my mind-set would have been if I didn't have O. J. Brigance in my life. He's always been there for me, and I'll always be there for him.

Like the biblical stories of Job, Peter, Paul, and David, O.J. has been tested and utilized by God. When you understand the trials that they all endured, you realize why O.J. is who he is and what really defines him as a person. When I see O.J. fight the way he fights every single day, I am reminded to live my own life right. In his presence, how could any one of us ever be anything less than our very best?

In just being who he is, O.J. inspires every life he touches, while impacting thousands of others. The work he and his wife, Chanda, do with the Brigance Brigade has advanced the quest for ALS research. And the job he's done with countless Ravens players as a mentor and role model over the years can't be quantified by numbers.

I hope this book speaks to everyone who reads it. I hope it gives you a reason to be your best self and pursue your dreams. When it hurts too much, or it just seems downright impossible, I always think of Juice and I find a way to keep going. I hope this book can do the same for you.

His spirit, his legacy, and his name will reign forever. Truthfully, it's hard to properly tell his story and express how he has inspired and touched the lives of so many people. His reach has been wide and there really is no end to his legacy.

I'm certain O.J.'s story is just getting started.

STRENGTH OF A CHAMPION

INTRODUCTION

IN life, you get a few special moments that you never want to forget. They're the times when you wish you could take a photograph that captures everything, eternalizing the entire scene, feeling, and essence of the experience. These moments rarely come along, but when they do, you have to seize them. You have to recognize them for what they are and savor every last second.

I had one of these special moments around eleven fifteen p.m. on Sunday, February 3, 2013. As purple, gold, and black confetti fell from the Mercedes-Benz Superdome rafters and covered me from head to toe, I wanted the moment to last forever.

The Baltimore Ravens, the NFL team that I'd spent the bulk of the last fifteen years either playing or working for in some capacity, had just completed one of the unlikeliest play-off runs in NFL history, rattling off four straight postseason victories after losing four of their final five regular season games.

After a dramatic 34–31 victory over the San Francisco 49ers, the Ravens passed the Lombardi Trophy from player to player, as kings of the football world. This remarkable group of men—

considered long shots to win it all by just about everyone—was now on the very top of the mountain. They were Super Bowl XLVII champions, an honor that nobody could take away from them for the rest of their lives.

As I sat in the end zone of the confetti-covered Superdome field with my wife, Chanda, I tried my best to take it all in, to remember *everything*. Seemingly every player and member of the Ravens organization came over and either hugged me or gave me a kiss on my head. One by one, I shared a glance, a smile, or an embrace with someone I loved. The mutual respect and admiration were real; the pulse of the team's collective heartbeat was palpable.

A former Ravens player and a member of the team's front-office staff since 2004, I have seen each and every one of these men come through the organization at one point or another. I've watched many of them battle adversity, on the field and off, as well as enjoy great successes. The 2012 Ravens, a group I often refer to as My Mighty Men, had just completed an incredible journey—both as individuals and as a collective unit.

For me, the Super Bowl victory marked a significant milestone in *my* life, one very few people thought I'd ever reach.

Five and a half years earlier, I was diagnosed with amyotrophic lateral sclerosis, or ALS.

I was just thirty-seven years old at the time.

A professional football player for twelve seasons and a Super Bowl champion with the Ravens in 2000, I'd battled adversity my entire career. Nothing I achieved in this life came without great struggle. I was born to teenage parents. With big dreams of playing in the NFL, I was lightly recruited out of high school. I was undrafted out of college. I played several seasons in the Canadian Football League before ever getting a shot with an NFL team. I overcame a back injury that was supposed to end my career.

I've been battling my entire life.

Though I didn't realize it at the time, all of those battles would serve as the foundation for my greatest bout yet.

I was diagnosed with ALS and forced to ask, "What now?"

Chanda, my college sweetheart and my Queen B, cried in my arms when we received the news. I cried with her. The weight of the diagnosis and possible outcome was hard for us to accept.

There were tears, frustration, and great pain.

Initially, I asked several questions. I wondered why and how this could happen to me—a strong, proud man who lived his life the right way.

It wasn't easy coming to terms with the reality of my situation. But each stage in life serves as a stepping-stone for the next. There are never mistakes in life, but learning opportunities. I came to realize that adversity is not only unavoidable, but necessary. Overcoming each obstacle strengthens us for new challenges ahead.

Our faith in Jesus Christ has enabled Chanda and me to keep a singular focus, no matter what comes our way. One of our favorite sayings is, "Life is a lot like school; there is never promotion without testing."

We've been tested.

We were told that most ALS patients live two to five more years after being diagnosed. They said there was a chance I wouldn't make it to my fortieth birthday.

But here I was in New Orleans, at the age of forty-three, getting showered by Super Bowl championship confetti and the collective love of the men and women around me.

I was a champion yet again.

I marveled at the moment, doing my best to savor every last image, every last laugh, and every last glance. I tried my best to take mental snapshots of the smiles, the joy, and that intoxicating taste of triumph. The road was by no means easy, but both the Ravens and I found a way to overcome adversity and reach our desired destination. Every day, we faced challenges—both as a team and as individuals—and we fought to rise above them.

Though ALS has robbed me of the use of my arms, my legs, and now my voice—I'm still here. I'm still fighting every day.

I can't walk, touch, or speak like I once did, but I believe that I am stronger now than I ever was before. As an ALS advocate, I am impacting lives more now than I did during my seven seasons as an NFL player. I still go to work every day. I still feel the rush of competition and see the fruits of teamwork and preparation. Both in football and in life, I see the goodness of man and the power of God every morning when I get out of bed. Through the Brigance Brigade, the foundation Chanda and I launched in 2008, we have raised close to one million dollars for ALS research and have affected the lives of thousands of individuals diagnosed with the disease.

I'm now six years into my bout with ALS, and I'm still making a difference in the lives of others. I'm still getting the very most out of all life has to offer.

I'm still here.

The toughest thing for people to understand about ALS is that I am still the same person and still have all my mental capacities. I can recognize you, so you don't have to introduce yourself every time I see you. I just can't talk or move.

Oh, and I am not deaf, so there's no need to scream. I can hear you just fine.

I heard those Ravens players and coaches just fine in the locker room after the Super Bowl. Ed Reed, a player I've known for more than a decade, was singing the lyrics to all of his favorite songs in his unmistakable voice. He'd just won the first Super Bowl title of his NFL career.

I heard Ray Lewis, my dear friend and a former Ravens teammate, tell me that I was his role model. He said I was his inspiration to keep fighting when he was rehabbing from an injury earlier in the season.

I heard quarterback Joe Flacco, a young man whose many critics believed he wasn't capable of winning "the big one," thank Ravens owner Steve Bisciotti for never losing faith in him. Joe was under the media's microscope in 2012. He could have crumbled under the pressure. Instead, he rose to the occasion and led the Ravens brilliantly throughout the team's play-off run.

I heard Torrey Smith, the young wide receiver with the engaging smile and a heart of gold, laugh up a storm. Torrey had been through an incredibly trying family tragedy earlier in the year when he lost his younger brother, Tevin, in a motorcycle accident.

I heard John Harbaugh, the finest of men, tell his wife, Ingrid, and his daughter, Alison, that he loved them.

I heard the sweet symphony of cheers and I heard the glorious sound of a collective goal accomplished.

I looked at Chanda, the love of my life.

It truly was the perfect moment.

Many of the Ravens players tell me that I inspire them. They look to my daily struggles with ALS and are lifted. The truth, though, is that those men inspire *me*. They have helped give me a reason to get up out of the bed every morning. There is a biblical proverb that says, "As iron sharpens iron, so one man sharpens another."

We are making one another better men.

Everyone has a purpose in life.

I've come to realize that the purpose behind *my* pain is to bring awareness to an orphan disease that is ravaging tens of thousands of people around the world. My primary purpose in the midst of my pain is to display how the light of Christ can illuminate a path to purpose in what would be perceived as one's darkest hour.

Would I have chosen ALS? No, of course not.

However, I have been given the opportunity to do my life's greatest work because I have chosen to fight and impact my circle of influence for God's greater good despite my circumstances. We all have a circle of influence that we can impact, no matter what the circumstances are in our respective lives. If you set goals and exhibit decency while seeking to achieve them, you will not only reap incredible rewards personally, but you will impact those around you in a positive way as well.

By the grace of God, I am blessed to get up every morning. I am still fighting. I am still loving life. And I am still fully capable of experiencing and recognizing those rare special moments when they come along.

We can't always control what God has in store for us. Inevitably, there will be obstacles, setbacks, and failures. That's life. But we *can* control our work ethic. We *can* control how we choose to approach whatever's next on the journey.

I may no longer be able to run a forty-yard dash like I once did, but I can still enjoy, cherish, and witness the best the world has to offer. I can still affect the lives of others around me.

I can still make a difference.

Six years after being diagnosed with ALS, I am still enjoying new experiences and achieving new goals. I am still getting up every morning and chasing my dreams.

I am still living my life to its very fullest.

I am no stronger than any other person. I've just chosen to make the most of every single day.

This is my story.

1.

THE KING OF KONG

What lies behind us and what lies before us are tiny matters compared to what lies within us.

—Author Unknown

I wasn't always the vocal team captain or the locker room leader. Though my former college, Canadian Football League, and NFL teammates may find this shocking, I was actually a very quiet kid while growing up in the Sunnyside section of Houston.

"Juice"—the introvert?

It's true.

I look back on my early childhood days with smiles and warmth, though it wasn't always easy being me. Long before I was "Juice," I was quiet O. J. Brigance, keeping to myself and avoiding interaction with people outside my family. When I first met my wife, Chanda, I was brimming with confidence—a college football star who thought he could do it all.

As a little boy growing up in Sunnyside, though, I wasn't full of *quite* the same bravado.

Sunnyside is located right outside the 610 loop and is just a few miles south of downtown Houston. It's the oldest African-American community in southern Houston and an area where family, God, and tradition are community staples. My childhood was marked by Sundays spent at church, family events, and block parties with friends from the neighborhood. Growing up in Sunnyside, we had everything we ever really needed. We weren't rich, but we didn't need to be. We had it all. We were blessed with friends, family, and fun.

I was shy and withdrawn, though, the result of a childhood speech impediment that kept me from being my true self. I would get nervous speaking in front of people and had a debilitating stutter. I literally had to stomp my feet to get the words out of my mouth in public settings.

I was embarrassed by the way I spoke and would often watch the other kids play from afar, fearful of the potential ridicule I'd face if they heard me talk. I opted to stay indoors, where I'd read books or play video games. While the other kids were out in the streets, playing tag or even causing mischief, I'd often be inside the house—playing Donkey Kong on my Intellivision video game system.

Donkey Kong was a great refuge for me at that time. I'd dive right into the game, envisioning myself as the Mario character, jumping around, climbing ladders, and earning high scores. People laugh or groan when kids say they love their video games, but I really relied on Donkey Kong at that age. It was a world of fantasy and fun. It was an escape. I didn't have to speak or interact with anyone. I could just be me, engaged in a sheltered universe of comfort and safety.

I was never really bullied in those days; it wasn't like that. Instead, I just avoided as much public interaction as possible. I was young—five, six years old—and I just didn't feel comfortable in my skin. The speech impediment kept me from being the "Juice" my friends and future teammates would eventually come to know.

I was a little boy, but I was already developing into a deeply introspective person. I thought a lot. I wrote things down. I prayed. I doodled. I dreamed. Looking back, I believe the speech impediment, as contradictory as it may sound, actually benefited me in the long run. It made me self-reliant. It made me use my mind in ways I'd never used it before.

It also gave me something I greatly desired to overcome.

As much as I loved playing Donkey Kong for hours on end, I wanted more. I wanted to live without fear. I wanted to join the other kids playing outside. I wanted to overcome my stutter.

So I did.

My family didn't come from great means, and in those days, there just wasn't the same access to speech therapists and pediatric experts that we have now. You worked through it with what you had. My mother came from a long line of strong, proud African-American women, and in her family, there was always a remedy for everything.

In the case of my stutter, my mother believed it was because I was an overly excitable child. Anytime I had to speak in front of strangers, I'd get animated, and rush to get the words out of my mouth. My grandfather did the same thing. Initially, my parents thought I was trying to mimic or emulate him with my stutter.

I hated my speech impediment. I just didn't know how to beat it. So we worked at it. And we worked hard.

Mom and Dad would tell me to breathe easy and to take the time to actually think about what I wanted to say before saying it. We'd do exercises on slowing down and processing all the thoughts in my head. "Think before you speak," Mom would tell me.

We'd spend hours reading words and enunciating. I eventually put down the video game joystick and repeated sentences aloud, looking into a mirror, instead.

With incredible support from my parents and the efforts of a few other very caring family members, I battled through my speech problems. They did drills with me whenever they could, back when they were all working other jobs and had their own personal hardships to overcome. Hard work, patience, and a wonderful support system helped me beat my stutter.

Eventually, I said farewell to Donkey Kong and joined the kids playing outside. In doing so, I discovered that I was a naturally gifted athlete. My ability to run and jump and throw—along with the newfound courage to speak without hindrance—gave me self-confidence that I previously did not know I possessed.

Ten years after those sunny afternoons spent inside my bedroom, too scared to play with the other kids my age, I was calling out plays from the offensive line for my high school football team on Friday nights under the lights.

Twenty years later, I was the face of a Canadian Football League team, doing interviews and appearing at community events every week in British Columbia.

Thirty years later, I was on a stage in a tuxedo, accepting the Johnny Unitas Tops in Courage Award, reading a speech to a room filled with hundreds of the most influential men and women in football.

It amazes me how by God's grace, I went from being a shy kid who once couldn't find the strength to get his words out to a public speaker and spokesperson.

Today, I serve as a voice for the thousands of ALS patients—my PALS—around the world who don't necessarily have the platform to reach others. My words carry more weight now than they ever did before.

That voice that you hear is technically not my own, but the words certainly are.

My childhood speech impediment was the first major obstacle I ever faced. With the love, support, and dedicated care of others, I conquered it. For all the many other things I'd go on to accomplish in this life, I could always look back to being the timid five-year-old-kid in Sunnyside, too fearful to say hello to a stranger, and know that I found the inner strength to overcome that.

I wanted to defeat my stutter and I did. It took patience, hard work, and the risk of embarrassment, but the end result proved that I could truly do anything if I put my mind to it.

I beat it.

As for Donkey Kong? I beat that, too.

Ask any of my old friends from Sunnyside; I'm pretty certain that I still own the neighborhood high score.

2.

WHEREVER YOU NEED ME, COACH

How much better to get wisdom than gold, to get insight rather than silver!

—Proverbs 16:16

WHEN I was playing football in the seventh and eighth grades, I always envisioned myself as Willowridge High School's next great linebacker. I loved the position. It's the only place on the field where you can run sideline to sideline, hit your opponent, and still call all the plays. The linebacker is truly the quarterback of the defense. Dick Butkus. Jack Lambert. Mike Singletary. These legends were the heart and soul of their respective teams. I wanted to be just that for the Willowridge High School Eagles.

After spending a summer bulking up working as a custodian at an amusement park in Houston called AstroWorld, I felt like I was finally ready—both physically and mentally—to lead the Eagles' defense from the coveted middle linebacker spot.

But God works in amazing ways, and sometimes life doesn't always go according to plan.

Prior to the start of my junior year of high school, John Pearce, the varsity team's head coach, called me into his office. We'd spoken only briefly before, and in my heart of hearts, I remember hoping he'd be sitting me down to tell me what I'd long wanted to hear: "O.J., you're going to be the starting middle linebacker on the varsity team this season."

Alas, the conversation didn't go quite the way I had wished for.

"O.J., have you ever given any thought to playing center?"

Center?

The center is the anchor of the offensive line. He snaps the ball to the quarterback and is expected to block the biggest opposing defenders at the line of scrimmage. It's by no means a "glamour" position, but it's arguably the most important one on the offense, outside of the quarterback. Look around the NFL and you'll see that many of the centers across the league are the smartest players in the game. The responsibilities are many, though any fame or glory is seldom.

I wanted to play linebacker. Butkus. Lambert. Singletary. Brigance! Now the varsity head coach was asking me about playing center.

"We're going to be running a different offensive scheme next year and we want to get smaller and faster on the offensive line," Coach Pearce explained. "We really need your smarts and athleticism out there. We want you to be the starting center on the varsity team."

In an instant, any visions of me gliding sideline to sideline or making a game-saving tackle on the goal line were replaced with a visual of me hiking a ball and getting bull-rushed by defensive tackles twice my size. I was considerably undersized for the position for the *junior* varsity level, let alone the varsity one.

I also was inexperienced. I began to wonder whether Coach Pearce was setting me up to fail.

I went home and told my father the news. He was surprised to see that I was disappointed. "You've worked so hard to make the varsity team," he said. "The coaches are coming to you with a great opportunity. So what if it's not the position you wanted to play? They obviously have their reasons. Go be the best center that school's ever seen."

Dad was right. Instead of viewing my new position assignment as a negative, I could view it as another challenge I'd overcome. In my fear and uncertainty around the position I'd be playing, I overlooked the wonderful news of the day—the coaches were coming to me and telling me they wanted me to be a starter on the varsity team.

Dad was a worker. His life was built around doing whatever it took to provide for his wife and kids. In this instance, he didn't see the negative. So I wasn't going to play linebacker. Big deal. I'd be on the field just as much, if not more, at center. Furthermore, he trusted that Coach Pearce and his offensive line coach, Coach Campbell, knew what they were doing. They obviously wanted what was best for their team. In this case, having me play center was just that.

The next day I knocked on Coach Pearce's door with an extra spring in my step.

"I'll play wherever you need me, Coach," I said. "And I can't wait to get started."

"That's great, O.J.," Coach Pearce told me. "You're going to love it. I promise. And you're going to be excellent."

I had the coaches' confidence. Now I just needed to learn how to play the position.

Fortunately, I had some pretty good players alongside me on the offensive line. Albert Jones was a six-foot-five-inch, 260-pound mountain of a man, and our right tackle. He could block anybody. He was one of the biggest kids in the school and everyone just called him "Big Al." Keith McDaniel, a five-foot-eight-inch, 210-pound road paver in the middle, played right guard.

My two best friends, Karl Lewis and Todd McQuietor, played left guard and left tackle, respectively. I did everything with Karl and Todd. It only made sense that we'd be lining up alongside one another on the offensive line. Even our numbers were in harmony: 57 (me), 77 (Todd), 75 (Karl).

I'd put our Willowridge Eagles offensive line up against just about any other offensive line in the state of Texas. Chemistry matters in football. And in the case of our group, we were always on the same page.

I quickly came to love playing center. In addition to touching the ball every play, I was the eyes and ears of the offense. If I saw a linebacker creeping in, I'd call it out before the snap for the rest of offense to take note of. If I didn't like the way the opposing defensive line was lined up, I'd make adjustments in the huddle.

Scoring touchdowns must have been thrilling, I'm sure, but I was having too much fun being the one blocking defenders and creating holes for teammates to really care.

When I was little, I always wanted to be Houston Oilers wide receiver Billy "White Shoes" Johnson. Though he was a fine player, White Shoes was best known for his flash, his style, and his elaborate touchdown celebrations. Long before Ray Lewis did his "squirrel dance" or Jacoby Jones was on *Dancing with the Stars*, Billy "White Shoes" Johnson was captivating the imagination of thousands of kids in Houston in the 1970s with his dance moves. I used to mimic his touchdown celebrations as a kid and wear my socks high up above my knees just like White Shoes. He was my favorite player.

Ironically enough, though, I played a position that was the

antithesis of everything White Shoes did. Centers don't score touchdowns, they don't get much of the spotlight, and they certainly don't dance. They do the dirty work.

I was beginning to realize that I was meant to be a center all along. After all, I was the kid who *chose* to spend his summers picking up garbage at an amusement park. Getting down and dirty in the trenches with defenders twice my size was right up my alley.

In truth, we all enjoyed those long afternoon practices almost as much as the "Friday Night Lights" games. We'd get after it with our starting defense and have spirited battles on the practice fields. The inside jokes, the memories, and the life lessons learned during those sweltering hot fall afternoon practice sessions remain with me to this day.

But schoolwork always came first, before football. Both in the household and in the locker room, academics always took priority. Coach Pearce had a "No Pass, No Play" rule: If you didn't pass your classes, you couldn't play on Friday nights. Other guys struggled week to week, but Todd, Karl, and I all made sure this would never be an issue for any of us. We took pride in our performance on the football field, but were even more diligent in the classroom. We all took honors courses and graduated in the top ten percent of our class. I'm as proud of that fact as I am of any of our high school football accolades.

Willowridge taught me how to have a voice and how to lead. I learned about teamwork there, and the pride of wearing the blue and silver. Our school motto was "Class and Character," and it defined the way we did things: with a spirit of excellence.

Toward the end of our senior season, Coach Pearce again pulled me into his office. Two years earlier he did this to tell me that I was being moved to the center position. Now he had something else he wanted to talk about.

"O.J.," he said with a bit of trepidation. "We think you can be a Division I college football player and we want to make that happen for you."

This was the elephant in the room throughout my senior year. I was having a great high school career as a center, but I was simply too small to play the position at the college level. Centers at Texas and Texas A&M were weighing close to 270 pounds. I was barely 190 pounds at the time. I had the grades and standardized test scores to get into some of the top schools in the nation, but without an athletic scholarship, attending one would be difficult.

I was chosen as the First Team All-State center in the state of Texas that year—a tremendous honor. Just about every other player on the All-State team was committed to playing major college football the following fall.

Aside from a few sporadic letters from Vanderbilt and Army, I hadn't really heard from *anyone*.

While teammates of mine were being recruited by Division I schools like Oklahoma, Houston, Texas A&M, Texas, and Baylor, I was widely ignored. Scouts from all of the colleges would attend our games and crowd around teammates like Jared Oliver, Big Al, and Charles Arbuckle after the final whistle. I'd finish a game and just head to the locker room. No recruiters were ever there to see me. I quickly came to realize that those letters of interest I was receiving were just pieces of paper.

The fact of the matter was that Big Ten, Big 8, Big East, SWC, and SEC programs simply weren't looking to give a scholarship to a 190-pound center—regardless of his accomplishments at the high school level.

Coach Pearce, though he'd never let me know it at the time, would later tell me that he hated the fact that I wasn't being heavily recruited. He saw qualities in me that he knew would shine at any level. He also knew what a gifted athlete I was. Playing center, I couldn't really show the college coaches my

4.5-second forty-yard-dash speed or my tackling ability. The position suited me well for Coach Pearce's offensive scheme, and it helped me develop important life skills, but it did me no favors as far as college recruitment went.

I have always believed that all I could ever ask for in life is an opportunity. However, if you give me the opportunity, the job is mine! At this point, I wanted to play Division I football because nobody in Division I football thought I could. It ticked me off, and I made a promise to myself that I would prove everyone who doubted me wrong.

Fortunately, I caught one man's eye. His name was Donald Dobes.

I was never going to play for the Texas Longhorns, but maybe—just maybe—I could play for Coach Dobes and the Rice University Owls.

Rice was best known as an academic institution, not a football one. People call it "the Harvard of the South." Though I lived just ten miles from campus, I'd never even been to one of their games. Truthfully, I wasn't even aware they had a football program.

Their head coach at the time was a man named Jerry Berndt. Coach Berndt came from the University of Pennsylvania and was looking for some intelligent, motivated young men to join his team at Rice. Donald Dobes, Coach Berndt's assistant coach, liked what he saw in me.

One day, Coach Pearce got a phone call from Mr. Dobes. He was calling to talk specifically about *me*. Rice was intrigued by my high school achievements, but knew I was too small to play center in the Southwest Conference.

"I never played him at linebacker, but I think he can be a great asset for Rice," Coach Pearce told the Owls assistant coach. "He's been playing out of position for me the past two years because I needed him to. He's the ultimate team player. He's got all the ability and smarts in the world to play linebacker in college."

Coach Dobes and Jerry Berndt were intrigued, but not entirely sold. Who was this kid who hadn't played a single down at linebacker in high school? If he didn't play the position for Willowridge, how was he going to be able to play it in college? They needed to see for themselves.

One afternoon, Coach Pearce told me to stay on the practice field long after the rest of the team had already gone home for the day. With the sun setting and darkness setting in, he brought me out onto the field, where there were a handful of coaches, all dressed in Rice University apparel, waiting for me.

"Show these guys what you've got, O.J.," Coach Pearce told me. "Go out and earn that scholarship."

With that, I was put through a personal workout from Coach Pearce. We did just about every drill you could imagine. For the first time since I was put on the blue and silver's varsity squad, I was being used as a linebacker. I showed my speed, I showed my strength, and I showed my smarts. Coach Pearce, in front of the Rice coaching staff, quizzed me on defensive schemes and linebacker positioning. I paid attention every day in practice, so I knew it all.

Colleges host NFL teams before the NFL draft and give their top prospects the opportunity to showcase their skills in things called "pro days." This was my "college day," and I auditioned as well as I could have ever dreamed.

After the workout, Coach Berndt asked me whether I'd be interested in playing linebacker at Rice University.

I thought back to that first meeting I had with Coach Pearce in his office two years earlier. I remembered my response at the time. I gave the same one to Coach Berndt.

"Wherever you need me, Coach."

I'd go on to play linebacker for the next four years at Rice.

I'd leave as the school's all-time leading tackler. I'm not sure whether any of that would have happened if I hadn't jumped at the opportunity to play center when it was presented.

Sometimes you've got to force yourself to see the forest for the trees. In that instance, just getting on the field was most important—not which position I was playing. Coach Pearce threw me a curveball in his office that day. After speaking with Dad and realizing that it was an *opportunity* and not a setback, I was able to hit it out of the park.

Life isn't always going to be easy. It's certainly not going to always go as you plan. The key is making the most of whatever detours you face. Not everything needs to be viewed as a negative. In many cases, the very circumstances you fear the most are the ones that turn out to benefit you in the long run.

Though I was initially disappointed by the new position assignment in high school, I eventually ended up playing linebacker after all.

I'd play the position for the next sixteen years of my life.

3.

SEEING THE LIGHT IN THE LOSSES

I think whether you're having setbacks or not, the role
of a leader is to always display a winning attitude.

—Colin Powell

THE day my parents dropped me off at the Rice University
dorms, I was a wide-eyed freshman with three specific goals in
mind.

1. I wanted to graduate.
2. I wanted to display the same "class and character" I
   prided myself on at Willowridge.
3. I wanted to play some football.

I'm proud to say that I achieved all of those things and so
much more.

I grew up at Rice.

I didn't know much about the school before I got there. From a football standpoint, the Owls were a program in transition. The longtime doormats of the Southwest Conference, Rice struggled against powerhouse teams like Texas and Texas A&M. There were no "pushovers" on the out-of-conference schedule, either.

It was as hot as fish grease during that first summer camp—so hot that we would get Popsicle breaks in the middle of practice. Growing up in the Houston heat, I was used to it. While some of the other freshmen were panting and gasping for air, I was thriving. I loved the conditions.

But playing defense was entirely new. I was a bull in a china shop out there. Our defensive coordinator, Coach Chismar, would affectionately tell me to put an anchor on my butt. I saw the ball go one direction and had no sense of what was happening around me. I needed to learn patience, and I was about to get a lesson through my first real injury.

I was notorious for shooting the back door on misdirection plays. This one particular time, I shot through the gap and dived to make a tackle. Fully extended, my leg bent awkwardly and I felt tremendous pain in my knee. The trainers came and checked me out, and it was later determined that I had a strained MCL. I would be out four to six weeks. For the first time in my life, I would have to miss a game. It was heartbreaking for me, but ultimately beneficial, because I was forced to sit, watch, and learn from the sidelines.

I learned more about playing linebacker from the bench than I would have had I been out there on the field like a deer in the headlights. I longed for my opportunity to get back into the lineup, but all of that studying helped me grasp the position. My knee was coming along slowly, and I was frustrated, but God just had me in a season of preparation for greater things to come.

When the knee was fully healed, Coach Berndt told me I

was ready. He also told me he'd never heard of a player making the transition from playing center in high school to playing linebacker in the Southwest Conference in a matter of five months.

"There's a first for everything, I suppose," he said with his usual wry sense of humor.

Coming back from an injury is always tough, because you not only have to heal physically, but you must overcome the mental hurdle to push through the pain and hesitation to get back to your old self. I primarily played special teams that season, until I got my first taste of game action on defense against the Arkansas Razorbacks.

IT was the fourth quarter and they were heading in for a score. Coach Chismar yelled, "Get in there, O.J.!" I ran onto the field with adrenaline pumping and butterflies in my stomach. I didn't squander the opportunity. I made six tackles in a little over three minutes of play, and we stopped them from scoring on the goal line. I barely remember anything from that night, because it was all such a blur.

After the game, the defensive coordinator of the Razorbacks came over and introduced himself to me. In a thick Southern accent, he said, "Son, my name is Fred Goldsmith. If I would have known you could have played linebacker like that, I would have tried to recruit you to play at the University of Arkansas. There wasn't any way that I could have gone to Coach Hatfield and said I have a hundred-ninety-pound center down in Houston that I want to play linebacker!"

We exchanged a few more pleasantries and parted ways after he put his arm around my shoulders and said, "You're going to be a heck of a player, son."

I had such a great sense of pride and fulfillment at that moment. At critical times, God will always validate our efforts to reassure us we are on the right path to our destiny. Coach Goldsmith reaffirmed that I had the talent to succeed on the Division I level.

Alas, we went 2–9 my freshman year. It'd only get worse from there.

My sophomore season, we went up against Arkansas again. We were 0–6 at the time and listed as thirty-point underdogs. The losses had been piling up, but we never got too down on ourselves. Coach Berndt kept our spirits high, and we were tied 14–14 late in the third quarter. The fans in Little Rock were getting antsy, wondering whether the home team was going to pull it out. I was making tackles left and right, and the rest of our defense was playing the best it had since I'd first arrived on campus.

A few minutes into the fourth quarter, we heard a collective gasp from the crowd. An "out of town score" had just come on the scoreboard. Number one–ranked UCLA, led by quarterback Troy Aikman, had lost to unranked Washington State. Word quickly spread to the field level, and we all looked around at one another in amazement. We were tied with the number nine–ranked team in the nation, and the following week we were scheduled to play number two–ranked Notre Dame.

Our focus was diverted. We all started thinking the same thing: *We're going to beat these guys, and then we're going to beat the number one team next week.*

Just as we started envisioning ourselves on *Sports Illustrated* covers and in ESPN highlights, Arkansas came right down the field and scored a touchdown. We lost 21–14. We played our hearts out, but we didn't keep our eyes on the prize. We looked too far ahead. The lesson there was to take care of what you've got in front of you. One game at a time. One day at a time.

We learned it the hard way.

Sure enough, seven days later we showed up to South Bend,

Indiana, ready to play the role of giant killers against big, bad Notre Dame. The weather was frigid, around ten degrees. It was early November, and we all piled on the layers of clothing in the locker room. Most of the guys, including me, had five shirts on. Despite our record, we were confident we could beat the Fighting Irish.

When we took the field, we looked across the gridiron at our opponents. There they were—Tony Rice, Chris Zorich, Raghib "Rocket" Ismail—some of the best players in the nation. And *none of them* were wearing sleeves.

I saw that and immediately stormed back into the locker room. There was no way I was going to be wearing five layers if my opponent was barely wearing one. I ripped off my undershirt, all the thermals, and left four layers of clothing on the locker room floor. My teammates followed my lead. If it wasn't too cold for the Notre Dame players, it wasn't too cold for us. "Hey, they put their pants on one leg at a time, too!" I shouted at my teammates, trying to motivate them the best way I could. These weren't some superhumans. They were college kids, just like us, regardless of our respective win-loss records.

We lost the game 54–11.

Though we fought valiantly, every week we left the field defeated. We didn't win a single game all season. We finished the year 0–11.

I was always a winner at Willowridge High School. At Rice, however, we struggled mightily. I would get so upset, because I knew how hard all the guys around me prepared each week and how badly we all wanted to win. We loved our coaches and wanted to win for them, too. Coach Berndt, Coach Dobes, and the rest of the staff poured their hearts and souls into our team, but we couldn't return the favor with victories.

Those long bus trips and plane rides home were always so quiet. I'd think about the games—every play—and want to linger on what went wrong. They say losing builds character. If that is the case, we gained enough for everybody.

"You need to lose a few times to really appreciate the wins," Coach Dobes once told me. "It's often the defeats in life that make the wins so gratifying. In life, it's important to see the light in the losses."

All those losses my first two years at Rice prepared me for bigger battles down the road. I'd fought hard and played to the best of my ability. Sometimes doing that results in victories, glory, and immediate gratification.

Sometimes it doesn't.

Through those lean first two years at Rice, I learned how to cope with defeat. There was no reason to carry a loss with you the rest of the week. It's okay to be disappointed for the first few hours, but you have to move on. Life is simply too short and too beautiful to dwell on the negative any more than you have to.

Losses are merely temporary setbacks. Nothing more. The key is how you get up and respond.

4.

THE ONE

Therefore a man shall leave his father and his mother and shall become united and cleave to his wife, and they shall become one flesh.

—Genesis 2:24

AS a kid, I always prided myself on being a gentleman. Though some of the other boys in my classes would tease me about it, I absolutely loved Valentine's Day. Every year I looked forward to February 14 as if it were Christmas or my birthday. A few days before the holiday, I'd take a trip with my mother to the local florist, candy store, and crafts shop. We'd buy all sorts of flowers, art supplies, and chocolates. When we got home from our shopping spree, I'd sit down at our kitchen table and begin working on thirty different Valentine's Day notes for all the girls in my class. Every single girl got one on February 14. I loved the idea of making all of them feel special on Valentine's Day.

I'm not sure whether it was because of the powerful presence of my mother, sister, and grandmothers in my life, but I've always been a sucker for romance.

I've never been too proud to say, "I love you," to the people I love.

Yet, by the end of my sophomore year of college, I still hadn't met a girl worthy of those words. I dated here and there throughout high school, but nothing really ever clicked. I was so absorbed in football and my schoolwork that I wasn't really courting any of my female classmates.

That changed a bit in college. I spent some of the money I'd earned at AstroWorld on a new wardrobe, and I drove a red Plymouth Duster. As a high school graduation gift, my mother's friend got me personalized license plates for my car that read, LEGIT.

Donald Bowers, my roommate at the time, saw my Duster with all its warts and bruises, noticed the license plates, and once asked, "'Legit,' O.J.? You sure you don't mean 'Leg it'? That thing doesn't have too many miles left on it. You'll be legging it soon enough."

But despite all the jokes and its critics, the Duster lasted me right through college.

I had the clothes and the car, but I still didn't have the girl. I was always looking for her, but as is often the case with the love of your life, I met her when I least expected it.

The summer after my sophomore year at Rice, Todd, Karl, and I went back to Willowridge to attend that year's high school graduation ceremony. We hung out on the top of the football stadium bleachers, saying hello to all the familiar faces and acting like the college big shots we now were. I knew just about everyone at the graduation except one person.

Sitting in a sea of people was the most beautiful girl I'd ever laid my eyes upon.

She glowed. "Who is *that*?" I asked my two best friends.

Neither Todd nor Karl had ever seen her before.

Throughout the graduation service, I was wildly distracted. I couldn't keep my eyes off of her. Who was she? Why was she there? What *planet* was she from? She was drop-dead gorgeous and carried herself in a graceful way.

Todd and Karl had long since moved on and begun to talk football, cars, and music. I couldn't pay attention to any of that. I was too busy staring at this beautiful girl in the crowd.

After the service finished, I was invited to a party at my mother's friend's house. I politely declined the invitation and headed home. I had to be up early in the morning for work, and I knew no girl at that party was going to hold a candle to the one I saw at the graduation ceremony.

As I got into bed that evening, the phone rang. It was my mother's friend Barbara, the host of the party. "O.J., you really should come on over. My goddaughter is here and you need to meet her!"

My mother got on the phone, too. "You've got to meet Barbara's goddaughter. She's beautiful and smart. You two would make a lovely couple."

When you're a single guy in your twenties, mothers tend to think *every* single girl they come across is beautiful, smart, and the perfect match. "Mom, I've got to be up early in the morning," I said. "I'm sure I'll meet her at some point."

I hung up the phone and shut off the lights. Then the phone rang a second time. It was my mother's friend Barbara . . . *again*. "O.J., you really should come back here and meet my goddaughter. Your mother and I are talking. You two are perfect in every way."

What didn't she understand? I had to work in the morning. Frustrated, I not only hung up the phone, but I put it off the hook. I needed to get to sleep.

Just as I did that, my cousin Lamont came barging through the front door. I knew he'd been at the party earlier in the evening. I called him into my bedroom and asked, "Did you happen to get a chance to meet Barbara's goddaughter tonight?"

Lamont's eyes lit up. "I didn't meet her, man, but she sure was pretty. Nobody introduced me because they were all saying how much *you'd* be her perfect match."

I responded, "Is she worth getting out of bed to go and meet?"

Lamont laughed and said, "Absolutely."

So that's what I did. I rolled out of bed, ran a comb through my hair, tossed on an old, dirty T-shirt, and shoved my feet into my muddy tennis sneakers. I hopped in the Duster, half-awake, and drove over to Barbara's house, where the party was still in full swing.

For someone who took so much pride in his wardrobe and appearance, this wasn't my shining hour. I walked into the house and there she was.

The girl from the graduation.

I couldn't believe it. My T-shirt was one the football team gave out that read, PRIDE AND QUALITY. It was two sizes too small and had a huge stain across the front. This was not the first impression I wanted to give.

I boldly approached the girl and introduced myself.

"I'm O.J. It's a pleasure to meet you," I said with my hand outstretched and my stomach in knots.

She looked me up and down and grinned.

"I'm Chanda," she replied. Then she followed the greeting with a question. "What's with the stained T-shirt?"

I let out a big, hearty laugh. She called me right out on it. I liked that.

We talked for a bit and hit it off. She was a few years older and studying at Texas Southern University. We came from similar hardworking families and shared a common interest in our hobbies and our love of friends. I asked her for her number that night, but she wouldn't comply. "I'm not real big on giving out my phone number to guys I just met," she explained.

I wasn't used to being rejected, so I didn't take her denial as a negative. I just figured I'd try again later. I asked my younger sister to ask Barbara's daughter Kandice for Chanda's phone number. After a few weeks, I got her seven digits and dialed her up. There was no answer, so I left a long, rambling message on her answering machine about how much I wanted to see her again.

She never called back.

So I tried again two weeks later. Another phone call, another message on the machine.

If she was trying to avoid me, she obviously didn't know about my persistence. I don't give up on things that I want!

I called her one more time. This time she finally picked up. I always consider myself a gentleman, but in this case I cut right to the chase.

"Hey, so, I've left a few messages on your answering machine and I haven't heard back from you," I began. "Let me ask you—do you or do you not want to go out with me?"

There was silence on the other end.

"Hello?" I asked, nervous that the girl of my dreams had already hung up on me.

"Nobody's ever spoken to me like that," she replied.

I'd blown it. I knew it. Before I could respond or apologize, she continued. "I have to admit I kinda like it. Sure, I'll go out with you."

We made plans for the following week. This time, instead of wearing a dirty T-shirt and beat-up sneakers, I wore a three-piece olive green suit. I'd bought it earlier in the week and thought it looked pretty sharp. I gave the Duster a wash, and I drove over to Chanda's place full of nervous energy.

When I got to her house and picked her up that night, she

looked beautiful. After she opened her front door, she again looked me up and down.

"What's with the three-piece suit?!"

From that point on, it was magic. I took her where my college student budget allowed that night—to the local Olive Garden. "Pride and quality," she remarked with a laugh, referencing the slogan on the T-shirt I wore the first time we met.

We talked for hours over dinner and dessert. She came from a family of athletes, including NFL star and former Willowridge alum Thurman Thomas, and wasn't impressed by the fact that I played football at Rice. She wanted to know what my dreams and long-term goals were. She wanted to know about my love of family and God. She was curious to get to know me for me, not O. J. Brigance, the college football player. I remember wishing the night would never end.

We continued seeing each other the rest of that summer, and when I got back to school in the fall, my training camp roommate, Donald Bowers, heard all about her. She was all I could think or talk about. Donald was one of my best friends at Rice, and the two of us always enjoyed going out together. "Am I losing my wingman, O.J.?" he asked me one night, with the look of a defeated man.

"I can still be your wingman," I told him. "But my 'playing days' are probably over."

God has a phenomenal plan. I have no doubt that seeing Chanda that summer evening in the crowd wasn't some sort of accident or happy coincidence. Despite both of our initial hesitations, God ensured that we'd meet. Once we did, we both knew we'd be together forever. I could have given up after my first phone call went unreturned. I could have walked away after the second. But sometimes you just *know* you can't quit. There are certain things in life—undeniable forces—that make you want to keep working, keep believing.

In the case of pursuing Chanda, the love of my life, there were no lengths I wouldn't go to, no sense of rejection I couldn't endure. Two decades later, I'm forever grateful that I didn't stop going after Chanda.

She's been my rock and my inspiration since that very first date. I love her and cherish her more now than I did even then.

And yes, I still own that olive green three-piece suit.

5.

NO DOESN'T MEAN NEVER

"For I know the plans I have for you," declares the
Lord, "plans to prosper you and not to harm you, plans
to give you hope and a future."

—Jeremiah 29:11

A new coaching staff was brought in prior to the start of my
junior year at Rice. As difficult as it was to say good-bye to
Coach Berndt and Coach Dobes, we all understood the nature
of the business. After a winless season, a change was in order.
Both men went on to coach at Temple University in Philadelphia, where they eventually got the wins and the respect they
deserved.

Of all the people in college football, our new head coach was
Fred Goldsmith—the same man who approached me after the
Arkansas game my freshman year. Coach Goldsmith didn't re-
cruit me out of high school, and I remember the motivation that

our postgame conversation gave me. He had an intense coaching style and had no problem being a hands-on teacher. I still had an underlying desire to show him that he should have recruited me, even though we were now on the same team and I was now playing for *his* Owls.

Under Coach Goldsmith, we went 2–8–1 my junior season. It was an improvement, but not by much. Toward the end of the fall semester, I was asked by our academic adviser to be a student career adviser for the Career Services Center. The purpose of the position was to encourage my fellow students to prepare for postgraduate life by participating in internships, and help them with résumé preparation. I really enjoyed it.

I was always intrigued by the types of jobs my fellow college classmates were pursuing, but I wanted to be an NFL football player. It was my lifelong dream. Working at a bank or in sales may have been more likely for me at the time, but even at that age, I always thought following my passion would make me happier than doing what the rest of society considered "successful."

Wisdom has shown me that if you do what you love, you will never work a day in your life. The Bible says it this way in Proverbs 18:16: "A gift opens the way and ushers the giver into the presence of the great." We all have God-given talents and gifts. Many times it takes life's experiences to reveal the gift. Rice served as my crucible to reveal the path for my life's journey.

My senior year, we turned things around on the football field. It was incredible. After three long seasons of devastating losses week after week, we put it all together and started to actually win some games. We were 5–5, heading into the final game of the 1990 regular season against Baylor. It was a week I'll never forget. For the first and probably only time in my four years at the school, everyone in the city of Houston was fixated on Rice football. We were one win away from our first season with a winning record since 1964. A victory over Baylor would not only put us at 6–5 for the year, but it'd give us an automatic bid into the Independence Bowl. Two years earlier we hadn't won a single contest. Now we were one victory away from playing in a major college football bowl game.

Coach Goldsmith had us all incredibly focused and prepared that week. We practiced hard and watched reels and reels of Baylor film. Minutes before the game, Coach asked me to address the team. I'd always been more of a "lead by example" kind of guy and wasn't one for rah-rah locker room speeches. I initially declined, but after some prodding, I stood in front of the locker room and spoke from the heart.

"This is what we've been working so hard for all season," I began. "It's what some of us have been preparing four or five years for. Win or lose, let's leave it on that field tonight. Let's never regret this moment. We never want to look back on today and think that we could have done more. We owe it to the fans to be our very best today. We owe it to ourselves."

The locker room erupted with cheers and we took the field, a team inspired. The game was a fistfight that went back and forth for four quarters. With a minute left, we trailed by seven points. The offense had the ball and was driving downfield, and I remember looking up and down the sideline at my teammates and then into the crowd. I made eye contact with my mother, who was seated with my father a few rows up in the bleachers. Mom smiled at me and shook her head in amazement. Of course it had to come down to the final minute. As she'd often tell me when I was younger, "Life's not always going to be easy."

Seconds later, we scored a touchdown. We trailed 17–16 with barely any time left on the clock. This was it. An extra point would tie the game, but it wouldn't be enough to catapult us into the Independence Bowl or assure us a record better than .500. Coach Goldsmith put up two fingers, signifying a two-point conversion attempt. I loved the decision. We were going for the win—leaving it all on the field.

Our quarterback took the snap and threw a pass into the end zone.

I held on to the hands of my defensive teammates as we watched the ball float in the air. With our mouths agape, we all followed the pigskin's flight as it fell to the ground.

Incomplete.

There'd be no bowl game or winning season. That was it. In a flash, it was all over. At that moment, it hit me—I'd never wear a Rice Owls uniform again.

Devastated by the loss, I watched as the Baylor Bears celebrated their victory on our home field. It was one of the toughest defeats of my life, but I'll never regret Coach Goldsmith's decision to go for the two-point conversion. He wasn't satisfied with a tie; he wanted the win.

It took days to get over the season-ending defeat, but when I finally did, it was time to look toward the next chapter of my life. I had aspirations to play on the professional level and expected to get the opportunity, because I had competed against some of the better players in the country. I finished my Rice career as the school's all-time tackling leader, the single-season tackling leader, a three-time Jess Neely Linebacker of the Year award winner, and a two-time All–Southwest Conference selection. I had the résumé to play in the pros and believed I'd be in the NFL the following year.

I began to train for my opportunity to work out for teams, but there was a lot less interest from the big leagues than I'd expected. A couple of NFL squads did come down to Houston to interview me. The interviews, however, weren't much more than a few questions and answers. I worked out for Jimmy Johnson's Dallas Cowboys, but never heard back from them.

For weeks I sat by the phone, waiting for calls from NFL

teams. The phone never rang. If there was one lesson that I learned behind the hedges at Rice University, it was resiliency. No matter what the obstacle, keep fighting. Keep believing.

Confused by the lack of interest, I decided to go talk to Coach Goldsmith to make sure he knew that I was interested in going pro and would appreciate anything he could do to help me.

To my surprise, though, he rubbed his hand over his mouth and began to compliment me on what an outstanding career I had achieved at Rice instead. His next sentence shocked me and made my pot boil.

He recommended that I take my degree and enter the corporate world. "O.J., you'd make a fine employee at a company," he said, dismissing my great desire to play football professionally. "You'll probably have a lot more success making decisions in the business world than you will in the NFL."

I didn't understand why he, my head coach and a man who knew how much I wanted this, would say something so discouraging. I respectfully said, "No, thanks, Coach. I will pursue my dreams to play in the NFL."

I remember leaving his office with the firm resolution that I would prove him wrong one way or another. I know now that he had my best interests in mind, but I couldn't see that then. He viewed me as a future CEO of a Fortune 500 company, not a professional football player. Though others would have been flattered with such an assessment, I was enraged.

Looking back, I see that Coach Goldsmith was probably as instrumental in my success as anyone. God allowed him to say exactly what I needed to hear to light a fire inside of me and to keep me from settling for anything less than what God envisioned for me.

His words served as a catalyst. On the wall in the coaches' offices at Rice there are lithographs of every player who made it to the pros—Tommy Kramer, Michael Downs, Courtney Hall, among others. For four years I passed by these pictures, imagining that one day my picture would be hung there beside the great players who had passed through the doors of Rice University.

The burning desire to be on those walls could not be extinguished by Coach Goldsmith or the NFL general managers who weren't dialing my number. I wouldn't let the dream die. I took matters into my own hands and called the one man I knew who also believed in my NFL dreams.

At that time, my old high school coach from Willowridge, John Pearce, had moved on to Texas A&M to serve as their tight end coach. I called Coach Pearce and asked whether he could get me into the Aggies pro-day workout, knowing there would be a large NFL contingent there. Coach Pearce had always been very supportive of not only his players, but players from Willowridge's rival high schools to help them get college scholarships. I knew he would have my back, and he arranged for me to work out with the Aggies on their pro day. Coach and his wife allowed me to stay at their home the night before. I called Chanda from their guest bedroom telephone that evening, and she told me I could do it. This was what we were waiting for—the opportunity of a lifetime. The next morning, Coach and I were up bright and early, headed to Aggieland. This was it.

I wish that I could recount a happily-ever-after ending from the tryout, but that just isn't my story. I didn't perform well and I ran mediocre times. Though men from twenty-eight NFL teams were in attendance, very few scouts stopped to introduce themselves to me.

Still hopeful, I watched the entire NFL draft on my parents' couch in Houston that April. Back then, the draft was twelve rounds, and 334 different college football players were selected. I stared at the phone that entire weekend, hoping I would get a call during the later rounds. However, the weekend came and went and the phone never rang. Not once.

I was confused. How was I not one of the best 334 players in college football?

I just knew in my soul that I could play on the next level. This is where God started teaching me, *No doesn't mean never. Just not yet!*

Some players take a direct path to the NFL. They are stars in college, get drafted in the first round, and are on the field the next year. But some players, myself included, have to endure a long and winding path before making it there.

My NFL story didn't end in Coach Goldsmith's office, on the Texas A&M pro day, or on NFL draft weekend.

In fact, it was just getting started.

6.

OH, CANADA

The road to success is always under construction.
—Arnold Palmer

I received a letter one day from the British Columbia Lions of the Canadian Football League, saying they wanted to come down to Houston and work me out. I initially dismissed the request, because I still had my sights set on the NFL. As the window for NFL training camp invites was closing, though, I thought maybe it was time to consider the league north of the border.

Canada might as well have been halfway around the world. I'd never followed the league and knew very little about it. A scout from the Lions—the B.C. Lions, not the Detroit Lions—named Bill Quinter followed up with me to arrange the private workout. Though the NFL was still my ultimate dream, I figured trying out for this CFL team couldn't hurt.

Realizing that I needed a better forty-yard-dash time, I worked for weeks with the strength staff at Rice to make sure my technique was right before my workout. The day came and I was ready to get the job. We had an evening workout scheduled under the bright lights of Rice Stadium.

Six p.m. rolled around and there was no sign of Mr. Quinter. Six thirty, seven, and seven thirty passed and he still had not arrived. I was worried that my last opportunity at playing professional football, even if it was in Canada, had stood me up.

Finally, my agent received a call from Mr. Quinter notifying him that his flight had been canceled due to inclement weather. He wouldn't be able to make it to the workout after all.

I was devastated. I'd worked so hard and had put so much positive energy into those weeks of preparation. I went back home that evening dejected and hurt.

Early the next morning, my agent called with incredible news. Mr. Quinter wouldn't be making the trip, no, but he *was* offering me a contract to play for the B.C. Lions anyway. I was elated.

All a man can ever ask for in life is an opportunity. As I always told myself, *If I get the opportunity—I will get the job.*

So off to Canada I went. Though I'm still slightly ashamed to say it, I had no idea where Vancouver was and definitely had never heard of Kelowna, B.C., where training camp would be held. I was thousands of miles from home, but I knew I had a job to do. God had me in the outskirts of Vancouver for a reason.

It was all part of the journey.

Though my surroundings were entirely different and I would go through temporary bouts of homesickness, I was at home the instant I put on those pads and stepped onto the football field. I had a solid training camp and eventually would be named a starter at inside linebacker. My first year in Canada was a learning experience, and though we weren't the best team in the CFL, I started to enjoy living north of the border.

My life changed forever during my second season with the Lions. That's when I met Danny Barrett.

Danny was a longtime CFL quarterback for the Calgary Stampeders and Toronto Argonauts. Prior to the 1992 season, our starting quarterback, Doug Flutie, left the Lions for Calgary, and we got Danny as our quarterback in exchange.

He was a fantastic football player, but an even better man. One day after practice, he suggested I grab some coffee with him. We started talking and immediately connected. Danny's football path was similar to mine. He was a very successful college quarterback at the University of Cincinnati, but was deemed too small to play in the NFL. He made his way up to Canada, where he made a fine living and had an illustrious career. He assured me that my experiences in Canada would open my eyes to just how expansive the world could be. In addition to being incredibly perceptive and engaging, Danny was also a man of great faith. He saw in me something few had seen before: He saw that I could share the gospel of Jesus Christ in a unique and impactful way.

"People listen when you speak, O.J.," he told me over coffee that day. "You have a gift. You can change people's lives with your words."

I'd gotten much more into my Christian faith during my time at Rice. I attended Brentwood Baptist Church near campus each Sunday. One day after a service during my sophomore year, a church mother named Mother Ball cornered me with a look in her eyes. She was known for winning souls for Christ, but I had no initial intentions of being her next recruit for Jesus. I was talking with friends when she tapped me on the shoulder and asked how I was doing.

I said, "Fine, thank you," and turned back around to finish my conversation, hoping she would move along to somebody else. She persisted, though, and pointed out how blessed I was to wake up that morning with clothes on my back and all my provisions met. She told me how fortunate I was to be able to walk and talk and be in my right mind. At that moment, it seemed like she and I were the only people in the room. I found comfort and inspiration in her words.

I attended church every Sunday morning as a kid, but up until that point in my life, I was more of an observer than a leader. Just like Mother Ball, Danny saw the light of God inside of me and thought I could do even more. He thought I could make a difference, and he took it upon himself to help me do just that.

We started meeting three to four times a week for something called "One-to-One Discipleship." Danny and I would go over scripture and he'd help guide me through different passages. He was a man of great faith and lived his life in a way I wanted to live mine. He also faced several setbacks and approached them in ways I'd never seen a man do before.

Danny's younger brother was a marine with a promising future when he was tragically paralyzed by a gunshot wound. Shortly after the shooting, he passed away in 1993, far too soon for a young man with such great potential.

Danny missed that entire week of practice. On game day, he said he wanted to play. We all dedicated the game to his deceased brother, but I couldn't imagine him being able to actually take the field. Danny—somehow, someway—found the courage to suit up that night. Not only did he start at quarterback, but he went out and threw for a record-shattering 601 yards and four touchdowns, leading our team to victory. It was an incredible thing to behold.

Danny was obviously devastated by the news, but I watched in amazement as he used the tragedy as an inspiration. He didn't lose his faith in God or question the reasons behind his beloved brother's death. Instead, he looked to God for guidance. Through his incredible devotion, Danny was able to find solace and community. He turned to his faith in a time of great adversity. In turn, he discovered the strength he needed to prosper.

His outlook on life was always so incredibly positive. I wanted the ability to approach every day in such a manner. He explained that most times, residual damage is self-inflicted, because when life's challenges come our way, we don't allow ourselves to wipe it off and move forward. Whenever I would hit a rough patch or obstacle in life, I'd reach out to Danny for perspective. He would often point to Romans 8:28, "We are assured and know that [God being a partner in their labor] all things work together and are [fitting into a plan] for good to and for those who love God and are called according to [His] design and purpose."

Danny's courage and devotion lifted *me* to new heights.

Slowly but surely, he brought me along in my Bible study. We started a gathering with some of our teammates that we called "the Men's Group," in which we'd all speak openly and honestly about life and our faith. Every player in that locker room had life experiences worth sharing with one another. Highs and lows—we laid them all out in the open with no judgment. We were all on such unique journeys, both in football and in life. Danny opened the doors to a whole new world for me.

During my second off-season, he convinced me to stay in Canada and work for an organization called Athletes in Action. We toured the country and organized high school rallies to spread the gospel across all of Canada. As I traveled, I would stay with a host family in each city. Various experiences in places like Saskatchewan and Edmonton helped broaden my horizons and grasp of other cultures. This was a growth period in my faith.

Danny and I played only two seasons together in British Columbia, but he's one of my best friends. He often calls me his "brother like no other." We had a saying that we'd tell each other over the years: "Press on."

When times get tough, press on. When you want to stop fighting, press on. When it seems like the hill is too steep to climb, press on.

To this day, every morning when I wake up, I think to myself, *Press on*.

7.

UNFINISHED BUSINESS

In their hearts humans plan their course, but the Lord establishes their steps.

—Proverbs 16:9

AFTER a breakout twenty-two-sack season for the Lions in 1993, I thought there was a chance the NFL might come calling.

It didn't.

Again, despite my accomplishments on the field in B.C., I was still on the outside of the NFL bubble, looking in. My agent, as frustrated as I was with the apparent lack of interest, said there was widespread hesitation about bringing in an undersized linebacker who was "already" in his mid-twenties. *Too small. Too slow.* And now, *too old.*

Chanda, whom I was dating long-distance all this time, and I prayed. I turned to God, citing John 14:1: "Do not let your hearts be troubled. You believe in and adhere to and trust in and rely on God; believe in and adhere to and trust in and rely also on Me."

I spoke at length with Danny about my situation, too. He had a wonderful fifteen-year career up in Canada, but never got his shot in the NFL. I was beginning to think mine wouldn't come either.

"You will make it to the NFL, O.J. You will," he assured me. "No doesn't mean never. It just means not yet. Your time will come. Trust me."

I had free-agent offers from multiple CFL teams that off-season, but felt good about a new CFL expansion franchise starting up in Baltimore. The way I saw it, for all the success I was having up in Canada, there would be more NFL eyes on me if I were playing in America. The more people watching, the better. Chanda and I discussed the opportunity and we both agreed it was the right decision. But I had something to take care of in my personal life before I inked any other contracts.

After the '93 season ended, I invited Chanda on a trip to Jamaica with me. We'd been all over North America, but hadn't gone on a real vacation since we'd started dating back in college. While at dinner one night at our hotel in Montego Bay, I convinced the waiter to put a blindfold on Chanda and present her with a special dessert. I got down on one knee, revealed a diamond ring, and asked the woman of my dreams to marry me over the sound of crashing waves and reggae music.

She said yes.

We had a very small wedding reception where both Todd and Karl gave memorable "best men" speeches. Since the moment I had first seen her, I knew Chanda was the one. We promised each other we'd always be there for each other. More than two decades later, I wake up to her smile every morning. It's my favorite part of every day. She is my everything.

———

I signed with the still unnamed Baltimore franchise in the spring of 1994. Chanda and I packed up my Ford Explorer, an upgrade from my beloved Duster, and made the twenty-three-hour drive from Houston to Baltimore.

Using the money we'd both saved up, we moved into an apartment in Owings Mills, a suburb a few minutes outside the city, and settled in as Baltimoreans. I knew Charm City was a great football town from the moment a few teammates and I went on a CFL caravan tour to promote the league's newest expansion team.

The city's response was electric. At a pep rally at old Memorial Stadium, the team unveiled its new uniforms and I served as the model, wearing number 94, signifying the year of the franchise's inception. After a short press conference, I walked the streets in my jersey and introduced myself to the fans. I loved their kindness, and the city embraced me as one of their own. That mutual respect and admiration hasn't stopped since.

I hit it off with my new teammates and we quickly took the CFL by storm. It's extremely rare for a first-year team to jell as fast as we did, but we all got along so well. Most of the guys on the squad, from our starting quarterback, Tracy Ham, to our star defensive tackle, Jearld Baylis, were veteran CFL players like me. We were fueled by our collective desire to prove wrong those who'd overlooked us over the years. Our coaches, led by the great Don Matthews, drew up offensive and defensive schemes that fit our personnel perfectly. And, man, we sure loved playing in front of our fans. They sold out Memorial Stadium just about every weekend. Aided by the fact that Major League Baseball was going through a strike that summer, we became the only show in town. Forty thousand people were showing up for Canadian Football League games. *In America!*

We went 12–6 our first regular season and beat the Toronto

Argonauts in a play-off game played in front of a raucous home crowd. The following week, we upset the Winnipeg Blue Bombers in their building. With the victory, we became the first American team to play in the Grey Cup, the CFL's equivalent to the Super Bowl.

The game pitted me against a very familiar foe. As fate would have it, we played the B.C. Lions in the championship game at BC Place Stadium. Many of my former teammates—guys I went to battle with for three years—were now lining up against me. To my amazement, thousands of fans from Baltimore made the trip all the way up to British Columbia to cheer us on.

I'd never played for a championship before, not at Willowridge and certainly not at Rice. This was *it*. This was my moment.

We led 17–10 at halftime. It was hard not imagining a parade through downtown Baltimore, but Coach Matthews did his best to keep us focused. Unfortunately, it wasn't meant to be. The Lions blocked a fourth-quarter field goal attempt of ours and the momentum completely shifted. B.C. stormed back from the seven-point halftime deficit and beat us 26–23 on a last-second field goal. As I did when Baylor beat us in the final seconds of my last game at Rice, I watched from the sideline as another team—my old one—celebrated the joy of victory.

The Grey Cup loss was a difficult pill to swallow, but the experience of a play-off run was exhilarating. The following off-season, we prepared to make a return to the championship game. We knew what it took to get there. The team came up with a motto—"Unfinished business"—and it became our rallying cry for the next twelve months.

Meanwhile, Chanda and I were growing to love Baltimore and everything the city had to offer. We walked around the Inner Harbor, made plenty of friends, and eventually even came to appreciate eating crabs, a Baltimore staple. We would marvel at the warmth and kindness we'd receive from everyone. If we were at a restaurant or a movie, there'd almost always be a fan there, waiting to pat me on the back or say, "Way to go, O.J.!" Houston would always be *home* to both of us, but Baltimore was making a very strong impression.

The 1995 season, my second in Charm City, was truly magical. Our team was now officially named the Baltimore Stallions, and we were a group of men on a mission. I had my best year with the team, earning All-CFL honors at linebacker, while serving as the squad's captain. There was a memorable road trip we took in which we played a game in Birmingham, Alabama, on a Saturday, followed by a Wednesday game in Edmonton, Alberta, and then Calgary, Alberta, on a Sunday. We were so focused on a goal that the weary week of travel didn't faze us whatsoever. We had a 14–3 record and were headed to the playoffs when we were dealt some alarming news.

The Cleveland Browns, a historic NFL franchise, were moving from Cleveland to Baltimore. This new Baltimore-based team would be starting up and playing games as soon as the following NFL season. The city's football fans were thrilled with the news—twelve years after the beloved Colts left for Indianapolis, the NFL was finally coming back to Baltimore—but we were left to wonder what would become of us.

We were told that the city's unbridled love for the Stallions was what ultimately convinced the Browns owners and the league that the NFL needed a team back in Baltimore. It was a small consolation.

The news was unsettling for many of us. We knew that with an NFL franchise coming to Baltimore, the Stallions would likely be forced to relocate. A lot of us had just settled in. Now, yet again, our lives would be in flux. A lesser team would have let the uncertain future derail it from its ultimate mission. We were not one of those teams. Knowing the end of the Baltimore Stallions was likely near, we used our "Unfinished business" motivation to lift us even higher.

We blew out Winnipeg and San Antonio in the play-offs en route to our second consecutive trip to the Grey Cup. This time, the game was played in frigid Regina, and the opponents were the Calgary Stampeders. They had the same 15–3 regular season record that we had and a starting quarterback whom I knew quite well—my old B.C. Lions teammate Doug Flutie. After short stints with the Chicago Bears and the New England Patriots, Doug ended up in the CFL, where he was the league's biggest star.

I looked at Doug, a former Heisman Trophy winner at Boston College, and struggled to understand how he was still playing in Canada. He'd won a Grey Cup for the Stampeders in 1992 and was the league's Most Outstanding Player. Yet here we both were all these years later, and he still hadn't been given another shot in the NFL. I realized that I wasn't the only one chasing the NFL dream. Even Doug Flutie, a household name in both Canada and the United States, was living his life on the NFL bubble, waiting for his chance. I had watched Flutie on the TV when I was in high school and learned from him when we both played with the Lions. Now he was the final obstacle blocking me from a championship ring.

The game went back and forth in the first quarter, and the Stampeders took an early 13–10 lead in the second. Coach Matthews rarely used me on special teams, but he called my number to go in and try to block a punt. "Wherever you need me, Coach."

The ball was snapped and I dived at the punter's feet, my arms outstretched. I blocked it! As the ball bounced around the field, I watched as a Stallions teammate recovered it cleanly and ran it in for a score. It was the momentum changer we needed. Up 17–13, there was no turning back.

At halftime, I made sure to remind the team that we led the previous year after two quarters, as well.

"Just getting here isn't enough," I said in another one of my rare attempts at a rah-rah locker room speech. "We need to finish the job! It is our time!"

We didn't squander any leads this time around, beating Calgary 37–20 in dominant fashion. I had my best game as a CFL player on the biggest of stages, recording ten tackles and blocking that punt. After the game, Doug Flutie came over and congratulated me. "Way to go, O.J. You deserve this," he said.

I'm happy to say that several years later, Doug did make it back to the NFL. He was a very successful NFL quarterback, right up until the year he retired in 2005, even making the Pro Bowl in 1998. Doug Flutie stuck with it. He just needed another chance.

In Canada, they treat the Grey Cup like hockey players treat the Stanley Cup. It's a beautiful trophy that gets passed around from player to player and is hoisted into the air. When I finally got the Grey Cup in my hands, I kissed it! We'd worked so hard the past two years, and I'd worked my entire life to be called a champion. That couldn't be disputed now. We finished the season on an incredible thirteen-game winning streak, and I had the ring to prove it.

I wasn't satisfied, though. Even in that wonderful period of great happiness and accomplishment, I knew the Grey Cup was merely a precursor to more that would follow. I was finally a champion, yes, but I wanted more. We celebrated with bottles of champagne and customized "Champs" ball caps on our heads, but I knew that night in the locker room that I would never play another down in the CFL. I was ready for the next chapter. I was ready for the NFL.

It was my time.

8.

PICK UP THE PHONE

Commit to the Lord whatever you do, and He will establish your plans.

—Proverbs 16:3

FOLLOWING our Grey Cup victory, we had a parade where we were celebrated as Baltimore's first champions since the 1983 Orioles. But it was all very bittersweet, as news would soon come that the Stallions' owner, Jim Speros, was moving the team to Montreal. I was once again a free agent and looking for a new job.

Don Matthews, my coach with the Stallions and now the man in charge up in Montreal, suggested I make the trip with him. I respectfully declined.

Chanda knew that for all of my success in the CFL, it was time for me to really pursue my NFL dream. She was no longer my girlfriend or fiancée. She was now my life partner. This wasn't just my journey; it was *ours*.

"O.J., if this is truly your dream, you have to do everything you possibly can do make this happen," she said one night as we discussed our future.

She was right. I wasn't getting any younger. I'd signed with Baltimore with the ultimate goal of having the NFL take notice. Perhaps it was all in God's plan to move the team and force me to take action. Chanda encouraged me to get out of my comfort zone and to create my own destiny. "You can't wait for the NFL to come to you anymore, O.J.," she told me. "You have to go and get it." I called my agent and requested that he make a real push to get me some tryouts.

A few days later he came through, and I was invited by the Cleveland Browns to work out for their team. The Browns, unlike the Stallions, mailed in the rest of the 1995 season after the news of their move became public. They'd be playing in Baltimore the following season and wanted to bring in a new cast of characters from top to bottom. Since I was already a popular player with the Baltimore fans from my days with the Stallions, it almost made too much sense that I'd play for them.

Chanda and I prayed the night before the tryout, and I arrived my usual fifteen minutes early. I was greeted by Scott Pioli, one of their young pro personnel assistants, and he knew all about me—from my days at Rice to my time in the CFL. I was feeling really good about everything that morning.

But I had an awful workout. I'd just completed a twenty-five-week whirlwind of a season where every other day it felt like we were in a new North American city. The Browns coaches put me through a bunch of drills, and I just didn't run well. I got tripped up in some of the linebacker tests and faltered on my sprints. Walking off the field that afternoon, I knew I hadn't displayed the best of my abilities.

My agent told me later that night that the Browns were going to pass on signing me to a free-agent contract. "It just isn't the right fit," they told him. I wanted to make excuses and pity myself, but Chanda wouldn't have it. I even considered calling Coach Matthews and asking about the opportunity in Montreal.

"You can't do that yet," Chanda said. "This team obviously wasn't part of God's plan. That's fine. So, what's next? We can't spend too much time lingering on the setbacks."

She was right. I had to shake it off. What was the point of sitting in the corner feeling sorry for myself? When I asked my agent for advice, he had few answers other than making a return to the CFL. That wasn't the solution I was looking for.

In the coming weeks, one of the league's two new expansion teams, the Carolina Panthers, told my agent they were interested, and we heard from the San Francisco 49ers, too. The Panthers actually made a contract offer, but later rescinded it for reasons I still do not know. It was devastating, but I tried to forge ahead.

Any visions of playing alongside Steve Young, Jerry Rice, and the rest of the 49ers were premature, too. Though I came in and had what I thought was a good workout, San Francisco never offered me a free-agent contract.

For five years, I waited for phone calls and workouts that pretty much never came. The few opportunities I did have just didn't seem to be coming through. Throughout my professional football career, I relied on others to find me and make my dreams come true.

It was time I broke out of my comfort zone and took a leap of faith.

During one of our many nightly discussions, Chanda insisted that no one could sell me better than me. There's a famous quote from the motivational speaker Michael Chitwood: "If you want something you have never had, then you have to do something you have never done."

I did just that.

I put together a list, in no particular order, of every NFL team. With the help of my agent and Mike Gathagan, the old public relations chief from the Stallions, I got the names and phone numbers of every head coach and general manager in the NFL. It was out of character, and something I never in a million years would have envisioned myself doing, but I decided to personally call every NFL team and ask them for a tryout.

Team by team I went. Team by team I was told, "No, thank you."

After personally speaking with twenty-five different NFL franchises and being rejected by each and every one, I considered giving up. Maybe Coach Goldsmith was right after all. Maybe the NFL just wasn't for me.

But Chanda wouldn't let me stop. "There are five more teams to go, right? Why are you stopping now?" she asked, pointing at the papers sprawled across our kitchen table in Baltimore. I thought back to something that my mother told me when I was younger: "Once you start something, you must finish it."

So onward I pushed. And on my twenty-ninth phone call, I got the response I'd long been looking for.

"O. J. Brigance?" the voice on the other end responded after I introduced myself. "The linebacker from the CFL?"

The man's name was Bob Ackles, and he was the general manager of the Miami Dolphins. As fate would have it, Mr. Ackles was once the general manager of the B.C. Lions. He started his career as a ball boy for the team. "I watched you play for three years while you were up in B.C.," he said. "You were one of the team's few bright spots. You had a nice little run with the Stallions, too."

Then he threw me a real curveball. "Jimmy likes you, too. He said he worked you out for the Cowboys back when you were at Rice."

I was floored. Jimmy Johnson had won a national championship at the University of Miami and two Super Bowl rings with the Dallas Cowboys. After working for Fox's NFL studio show for a few years, he was the new head coach of the Miami Dolphins. I'd watched Jimmy Johnson coach winning teams on TV for most of my adult life. My tryout with the Cowboys five years earlier was a less than memorable one. Jimmy Johnson knew who *I* was?

"So, you're looking to play in the NFL now?" Mr. Ackles asked rather casually.

"Yes, sir," I answered. "I just finished my fifth season in the Canadian Football League and am currently a free agent. I want to be a Miami Dolphin."

Bob Ackles didn't laugh, as some of the other general managers and coaches I called had. He responded with the only thing I ever needed in this life—a chance.

"I'm going to ask you one question, Brigance," he said. "Can you run a forty-yard dash under four-point-six seconds?"

My tongue was quickly tied. I faced a dilemma on this one. The truth of the matter was that I hadn't run a forty-yard dash in under 4.6 seconds since college. But I wasn't going to say no. Without much hesitation, I replied, "Yes, sir. I can run a forty-yard dash under four-point-six seconds. No problem."

Sometimes you have to step out in faith! I not only stepped out, but took a giant leap on that one. Mr. Ackles then asked me what I thought my former head coach with the Stallions, Don Matthews, would say about me.

"He would say that I am a good linebacker and a very good leader both on the field and off," I replied. Mr. Ackles had a long history with Coach Matthews and said that he'd call me back in the coming days after he spoke with him. I thanked him for taking my phone call, and he thanked me for being proactive and reaching out.

I put the phone down and ran over to Chanda, who was in the next room. It wasn't anything to celebrate yet, but after my being rejected twenty-eight times in a row, this was certainly a step in the right direction. We were both very excited and knew that Coach Matthews would only speak highly of me.

Then she said something that showed just how committed to this cause she was. "You still have one more team to go, right?"

I did. I called the Houston Oilers, my hometown team and the franchise I grew up rooting for. To my great surprise, the Oilers were interested in bringing me in for a workout, too. Their general manager, a man named Floyd Reese, had scouted me back when I was at Rice. We spoke briefly and he said he'd be in touch shortly.

After twenty-five straight nos, two of the last teams on my list were interested. I'd wanted to give up after twenty-five. My mother used to always say, "If you're going to start something, you'd better be willing to finish it. Otherwise, what's the point?"

I had wanted to give up prematurely, despite this lesson from my mother, but Chanda wouldn't allow it. I'm incredibly grateful to both of them for staying the course when I began to falter. It helps having two incredibly strong-willed women in your life. I learned then, as I would several more times in the future, that it's *imperative* to see things through to completion.

As Chanda and I sat astounded by the positive turn of events in our living room, the phone rang in the kitchen. It was Bob Ackles from the Dolphins. He had already spoken to Coach Matthews.

"When it comes to football, there are few opinions I trust more than Don Matthews's," he began. He then followed up with a question I'd been waiting years to hear: "Can you be on a flight this afternoon?"

"Yes!" I responded. The flight was booked and I was headed to South Florida.

Before I left for the airport, though, the phone rang again. It was the Houston Oilers. They wanted to sign me to a contract without my even working out for them. After so much rejection and heartache, one team was flying me in to meet with them and the other was offering me a free-agent contract.

The situation in Miami just felt right. I thought the Cleveland Browns one did at the time of my workout, but it really didn't. The Browns didn't know me and I didn't know them.

The Dolphins were starting anew and so was I. Don Shula, their longtime coach of twenty-six years, had just retired, and Coach Johnson was coming in as the new headman. With him would come a new atmosphere, new style, and some new players. I desperately wanted to be one of those chosen few.

I flew down to Fort Lauderdale and stayed in the team hotel. I called Danny Barrett on the telephone the night before. We prayed together and discussed the following morning's tryout. We agreed that if Danny wasn't going to make it to the NFL, at least one of us would. He was as determined that I'd make the most of my Dolphins opportunity as I was. This wasn't just my chance. It was *ours*.

I worked out for Coach Johnson and his staff in the blazing South Florida heat. George Hill, the defensive coordinator, had me running wind sprints sideline to sideline. Because of the different field dimensions in the CFL, this wasn't a problem for me. I ran like the wind.

Then came the moment of truth: the forty-yard dash.

I'd probably run "the forty" a thousand times in my life. I hadn't cracked 4.6 seconds in about five years. Lining up for the sprint, with all of the Dolphins coaches and scouts and their stopwatches staring back at me, I could feel a giant pit in my stomach. I took a moment before I got in running position and prayed, "God, I am really out here now and need you to back me up. Please, Jesus!"

As I got into my stance, I continued praying, saying aloud, "Do it, Lord! Do it, Lord!" I exploded from the start and was digging with all I had inside of me. I felt like a bolt of lightning as I ran through the thick, humid South Florida air. I finished through the line, heard all the stopwatches beep, and ran another fifteen to twenty yards down the field. I stopped with my back to Coach Hill and screamed, "Please, Lord, make it happen!"

I turned and looked straight at Mr. Ackles, the man I told I'd be able to run the forty-yard dash in less than 4.6 seconds one day earlier. I'll never forget his response, as it was the opening of the gates to the NFL for me. He looked my way and gave the slightest head nod and smile.

"Four-point-five-seven," said one of the scouts.

Four-point-five-seven! I did it!

"Do it, God!" I screamed aloud.

After the workout, I introduced myself to Coach Johnson. "Of course I remember you," he said with his familiar Texas accent. "You boys at Rice beat my Arkansas Razorbacks a few years back, much to my dismay. You were all over the field that day, Brigance."

Someone was watching those games after all.

Whereas my Browns tryout a few weeks earlier hadn't gone as I had hoped, I felt as if I were on top of my game in front of all of the Dolphins' key decision makers, and loved meeting with Coach Johnson. He wasn't as concerned with the size of the dog, but the fight in the dog.

Later that afternoon, Mr. Ackles offered me a free-agent contract to join the Miami Dolphins. I'd have to make the team in training camp, but my NFL opportunity was finally granted. As I always told myself, *If I get the opportunity—I will get the job.*

There was no way I wasn't getting this job.

Chanda and I celebrated with tears of joy when I shared the

news with her that evening. We'd prayed for this chance for so long, and now that it'd finally arrived, we both knew that I would make the very most of it. I called the Oilers back and shared with them my decision. They said they understood and wished me the best of luck.

Whenever kids ask me what they can do to land an interview for their dream job or get the big internship they want, I tell them the honest truth: Pick up the phone. The opportunity might just be a phone call away.

9.

JIMMY'S WORLD

I run on the road, long before I dance under the lights.
—Muhammad Ali

I showed up to Dolphins training camp that July in the best shape of my life. Coach Johnson was originally from the college ranks, and his approach to practice may have surprised some of the longtime NFL veterans. We went at it in full pads and were expected to go full speed. In some NFL training camps, the coaches take things slow and cater to the team's bigger stars. Not in Jimmy Johnson's. I arrived as an unknown Canadian Football League journeyman and was treated the same as Dan Marino. We were all expected to give it our all and never let up. I'd have it no other way.

From the beginning, Coach Johnson made his intentions and priorities crystal-clear. In his first team meeting, he said, "Men, I am a selfish SOB! If you can help me win, you will be on this team. But if you can't, you can be my best friend and I will cut your tail!"

He wasn't kidding. Though it sounded harsh, I saw hope in his statement. I heard, "If you perform, you will be here."

But when we got to work that July, it hardly looked like I would get the job. I was sixth on the depth chart at the linebacker spot at the start of camp. Linebackers usually wear numbers in the fifties, but I was given number 45, because there were already too many uniforms in the fifties handed out. I tried not getting too down, telling myself that there was nothing to lose and nowhere to go but up.

I turned to one of my favorite biblical passages, from Hebrews 11:1: "Now faith is confidence in what we hope for and assurance about what we do not see."

To achieve all God has in store for us, we must believe in ourselves even when the circumstances seem stacked against us.

It may have looked like a long shot on paper, but life isn't lived on paper. *Especially* not a football life.

I went to work controlling what I could control—my work ethic and attitude. It was time to compete. It was evident very quickly that this was a different level from the competition I faced in the CFL. I was running with fullback Keith Byars step for step and knew I had him covered on a seam route. The next thing I heard was a quick whistle whiz by my ear. Seconds later, Byars was in the end zone with the football and I was ten yards behind him, wondering what had happened. That quick whistle was the football, thrown by Dan Marino. It was a perfect back-shoulder fade pass, one that I'd never seen—or heard—completed before. I looked at Marino in disbelief and he gave me a devilish grin that was his competitive trademark. It was as if the pass were Marino's way of saying, "You aren't in Kansas anymore, Dorothy!" Or better yet, "Welcome to the NFL, kid."

After the first day of practice, I noticed a soda machine in one of the hallways of the team facility in Davie, Florida. I was ten cents short of the usual fifty cents it cost to get a can of soda, so I asked a few of the veterans whether they could spare a dime. One by one I went, and at least five of them just shrugged their shoulders with quizzical looks. Dwight Hollier, a fellow linebacker who'd been in the NFL for five years at the time, did me a favor and pulled me aside. "This is the NFL, man," he said with a laugh. "You don't have to pay for sodas."

It was all so new to me. When I first got to the CFL, I had to pay for my own gloves and shoes. I never even thought twice. The NFL was really the big leagues, from suiting up alongside legends like Dan Marino to perks like free cans of soda.

But there was nothing cushy about that summer. Training camp under Coach Johnson was downright brutal. We practiced in one-hundred-degree heat in the morning and we were instructed to tackle to the ground. We wore shoulder pads and shorts in the afternoon. This was supposed to be a "thud" session, which meant we'd go full speed to the point of contact and then wrap up instead of tackle. That didn't last very long. By the second week of camp, we were hitting one another in the afternoons, too.

My first affirmation that I was catching the eyes of the coaches came from Coach Johnson himself. We were in a seven-on-seven drill and running back Terry Kirby ran an out route toward me. I broke on it perfectly and knocked the ball away with my play-side hand. Textbook. I jumped up enthusiastically and pumped my fist. Coach Johnson jogged over and said, "Brigance, if you keep making plays like that, you will make this team!" I was already motivated. Those words just threw fuel on the fire. I thought to myself, *All things are possible with God!*

During one of our first days of training camp, an undrafted rookie linebacker introduced himself to me on the practice field. "You're O. J. Brigance, right?" I recognized his face, but couldn't quite place his name.

"I'm Larry Izzo," he said with a smile. "I played linebacker at Rice after you left. You're a legend, man."

That's how I knew him! After I graduated, Izzo carried the torch and led Rice to their long-awaited winning season. He was a standout at the collegiate level but, like me, went undrafted. He, too, was trying out for the Dolphins. Izzo wasn't the fastest or strongest guy in training camp that summer, but he was a fighter. And in Jimmy's world, fighters always stood a chance.

In addition to Larry Izzo, there was another rookie linebacker who demanded everyone's attention. His name was Zach Thomas, and he had a motor that didn't stop. Drafted in the fifth round out of Texas Tech, he was another guy, like both Larry and me, who was deemed "too small" to make it in the NFL. Other teams passed on all of us. We were determined to make them all regret it.

Larry, Zach, and I became fast friends. I was considerably older—in football terms, at least—than both of them, so I took on a bit of a big-brother role. There was no guarantee that any of us would make the team, but we all had outstanding training camps. I'd waited my entire life for this opportunity. Larry and Zach wanted it just as badly.

One afternoon, we played Norv Turner's Washington Redskins in a scrimmage. Coach Johnson and Coach Turner had a long history of coaching together with the Super Bowl–champion Cowboys, but this scrimmage was anything but friendly. After a play in which he thought he was given a cheap shot, Larry got up and went after a pack of Redskins players. He took on four of them, pushing, shoving, and calling them every name in the book. We broke up the scrum and Larry staggered back to the sideline, panting like a dog. He had scratches all over his face. "Let me back out there!" he shouted to no one in particular. It was just a training camp intersquad scrimmage, but Larry was treating it like the Super Bowl. I loved his spirit, but not everyone on the team was thrilled with his reaction. Some of the veterans on the team rolled their eyes and told him to calm down.

Later that night, Coach Johnson called Larry out in front of the entire team at our evening meeting. I feared the very worst. Knowing Coach Johnson, there was a chance that he would cut Larry right then and there. He had no problem sending players home at the drop of a dime.

"Izzo!" he yelled. "Where are you from?"

Larry, a bit scared by the question, responded, "Woodlands, sir!"

"Outside Houston, right?" asked Coach Johnson.

Larry nodded.

"Good! Well, you call your family out in Woodlands, Texas, and you tell them that only two guys have made the 1996 Dolphins roster right now—Dan Marino and Larry Izzo!"

That was Coach Johnson. There were Pro Bowlers and veterans at every position, but because Larry was giving it his all and treating an intersquad scrimmage like it was the Super Bowl, only he and Marino, an eventual Pro Football Hall of Famer, were deemed "locks" to make his squad. The statement sent a message to the rest of the team. It inspired me to play even harder and faster.

It was tough *not* to want to give it your all for a coach who rewarded hard work and dedication. Coach Johnson cut long-time veterans on the spot if they were dogging it, and didn't care what college you attended or how fast you ran a forty-yard dash at the NFL draft Scouting Combine. That summer he released Dorian Brew, the team's highly decorated draft pick out of Kansas, because he wasn't picking the defense up fast enough. No one's job was safe. Jimmy wanted players who'd give it their all and leave everything on the field. Your résumé on paper carried no weight with this man if you didn't fit his plan.

A few weeks into the 1996 preseason, the Dolphins cut the roster down from ninety players to seventy-five. I was one of the seventy-five still left standing. Then they cut it down to sixty. I was still there. Over Labor Day weekend, they announced the final fifty-three-man roster.

In big, bold letters right at the top of the list, I read what I'd been dreaming to see for years: "O. J. Brigance, Linebacker."

I'd finally made it to the NFL.

God took me on the scenic route, but I eventually got there. The people who said I couldn't? They didn't determine my destiny.

Proverbs 3:5–6 says, "Trust in the Lord with all your heart and lean not on your own understanding; in all your ways submit to him, and he will make your paths straight."

In addition to Larry and me, Zach made the team as well. The three of us had lockers next to one another and lived by a shared edict: "Give it all you've got." We were beyond grateful to just make it to the NFL, but knew that wouldn't be enough to sustain long NFL careers. We'd have to treat every play as if it were our very last.

Larry and I became key cogs on the Dolphins special teams unit, chasing down punts and kickoffs like our lives depended on it. And whenever needed, I would jump in at linebacker and rush the quarterback. Coach Johnson once asked me whether I was willing and able to play safety, if needed.

"Wherever you need me, Coach." That mantra had worked for me in the past. Fortunately, I was never asked to play the position. I would have been lost!

As Larry and I did our thing on special teams, Zach flourished as a starting linebacker, earning All-Rookie honors and a Pro Bowl nod in his first year. Though I had a few years on him, I learned a lot from Zach. When we'd watch game tapes, he would write down the formation and play and the number of times the team would run it in their offense. He taught me an organized way to study film.

We were three guys from Texas, cutting our teeth together in the big leagues. With both of their families living so many miles away, Chanda and I hosted Larry and Zach for dinners during the holidays every year. In the NFL, you come across hundreds of teammates. Guys come and go. Larry and Zach were more than teammates, though. They were my brothers.

Larry would go on to win three Super Bowl rings with the New England Patriots and make the NFL's All-Pro team three times as a special teams standout. Zach played fourteen years in the league and was picked to go to the Pro Bowl in Hawaii seven times. He was named to the 2000's All-Decade team as one of three starting linebackers. All three of us enjoyed long NFL careers. To this day, we all look back on our time spent together in Miami, when we entered the league as three long shots to make the team, as the critical foundation to each of our eventual successes.

10.

DOLPHIN DAYS

Energy and persistence conquer all things.
—Benjamin Franklin

THE Dolphins went 8–8 and missed the play-offs in 1996. I played primarily on special teams and tried to make a difference where I could when used at linebacker. On the field, I played well, but knew I could do more. Off the field, I worked to make a difference in the community and with the team. Chanda and I devoted ourselves to multiple community organizations and causes, including Habitat for Humanity, the Cystic Fibrosis Foundation, and the Daily Bread Food Bank. I found as much joy in fighting for these causes as I did in taking on opposing blockers.

I also found a few guys on the team who were as devoted to their faith as I was, and helped organize a group Bible-study session. We met a few times a week and kept it relatively loose.

Teammates could drop in here or there, or come every time we met. It was a great outlet for all of us and a wonderful way to build our trust.

A wide receiver named Qadry Ismail joined the Dolphins prior to the start of the 1997 season. On one of his first plays of practice, Qadry came running across the middle on a slant pattern and I popped him right in the mouth. It was a clean hit, but a devastating one. I knew what Jimmy Johnson wanted to see from his linebackers in practice, and that was full-speed contact, even in August. Qadry got up slowly from the blast and was visibly shaken. When he finally came to, he had a look of rage in his eyes. He was looking to fight me right then and there on the practice field. I wasn't one for fighting teammates, and I did what I always did when an opposing player came at me—I just smiled back at him. Kill 'em with kindness! Qadry muttered something under his breath and shuffled back to the huddle, a bit dazed.

A few weeks later, I noticed Qadry hadn't made too many friends on the team, and I wanted to reach out. From a professional standpoint, our offense and special teams unit needed him to succeed. From a personal one, I didn't like seeing a teammate feel as if he were on the outside.

I invited Qadry to the Bible-study group that I was leading and assured him that he wouldn't be expected to speak or contribute if he didn't want to. He respectfully declined my invitation and went about his business. That was fine by me, as long as he knew the invitation was there.

One afternoon that September, though, I was pleasantly surprised to see a new face in our group Bible-study session after practice. It was Qadry. He sat in the back and didn't say much at first, but as he continued to attend our meetings in the coming weeks, he began to open up. Toward the end of the season, Qadry had become one of the more popular guys in our "Men's Group." The bond he felt in our Bible-study sessions was something he had long craved. As he felt more comfortable with us off the field, he began to perform better on it.

I'd later be teammates with Qadry in Baltimore, where he would often *lead* the team's Bible-study sessions. As a Raven, Qadry was a much different person than he was in his first days as a Dolphin. He'd matured and grown—both as a football player and as a man. Qadry's still a dear friend of mine to this day. After his playing career was finished, he needed to undergo neck surgery at Johns Hopkins Hospital in Baltimore. Chanda and I hosted his wife, Holly, and their three children in our home during that anxious time in their lives.

Qadry, meanwhile, has always been there for me. He now serves as a radio analyst for the Ravens. Not a week goes by that Q doesn't drop by my office and check in on me, my state of mind, and my spirit. He asks how Chanda is doing and he asks how he can *help*. Q's my brother.

It's amazing to think that we very nearly came to blows the first time we met.

The Dolphins went 9–7 in 1997, losing in the wild-card round of the play-offs to the rival New England Patriots, 17–3. The loss was especially hard because of the way we finished the season. After jumping out of the gates 5–2 and atop the AFC East division, we lost our final three games of the year, including an embarrassing 41–0 loss to the Colts in week fifteen. The late-season swoon affected us all, but no person more than Coach Johnson. He was a winner with the Miami Hurricanes and with the Dallas Cowboys and didn't like the way we'd closed out the campaign. "You have to finish the job," he told us. "You can't kick back and assume everything will work itself out fine. You need to go out and make sure it does."

Though we were different men in many ways, Coach Johnson and I lived by a similar code: Life doesn't just come to you. *You have to go out and get it.*

We bounced back in 1998 and once again made the play-offs.

After beating the Buffalo Bills in the wild-card round, though, we lost to the Broncos in their building, 38–3. Denver would go on to win the Super Bowl a few weeks later. For us, the play-off loss in Mile High Stadium was a devastating defeat and made for yet another heartbreaking end to the season. As the special teams captain and one of the leaders in the locker room, I tried offering some words of encouragement, but couldn't find the right thing to say. We'd have to make another go of it the next season.

But there almost never *was* a next season for me.

One day while participating in the off-season voluntary workouts preceding the '99 season, I felt an excruciating pain in my lower back. I tried to fight through it like I had with injuries in the past, but this pain was different. I experienced numbness in my right leg and my foot just dropped. I couldn't flex my foot, and it scared me because I didn't know what was going on.

The Dolphins trainers checked me out, determining that I needed to get an MRI done. In the meantime, I started doing exercises to try to strengthen my back, but nothing worked. It was painful to bend over to brush my teeth or sit down or stand. My walk was restricted, so I kind of waddled along everywhere I went. I wasn't myself.

Our team doctor referred me to a back specialist at Jackson Memorial Hospital in Miami. From the time I left the practice field, through the entire rehab process, I kept praying that God would make it all right.

We all have experienced déjà vu at some point in our lives. In a dream, I saw my doctor visit before it occurred. I saw myself in the doctor's office sitting across the desk from him. He looked at the MRI and said, "There is a chance that you have played your last down of football."

In the dream, God said to me, "Don't believe him. Prepare for and have the surgery. It will all be okay!"

This all occurred before I ever went to the appointment. Days after my vision, I went for my MRI and it revealed stenosis of my spinal canal in my lumbar area. The restriction was squeezing my spinal cord, causing the pain and numbness. It was time for my consultation to discuss the results. I was stunned as the consultation played out exactly as it had in my dream. I sat there as the doctor said verbatim what had been revealed in my vision several nights earlier.

When he got to possible options to fix the stenosis, he explained that during the surgery, they would go in and widen the spinal canal at the restricted area. This process, he warned, would be extremely sensitive and would take seven to eight hours to complete.

The doctor said, "Hopefully we can get you back to walking normally, pain-free. However, there's a chance you won't be able to ever play football again."

As he was explaining everything, I sat there with a slight grin on my face, because I had already received confirmation that everything would be all right! Once the doctor laid out all the options, he advised me to take some time to think about what I wanted to do.

I didn't need to think it over, because I knew I was already healed. God had assured me that I'd be all right. I said, "Let's schedule it," without much hesitation at all.

The day of my surgery came and I was quietly confident, singing my favorite gospel song as I went into surgery, Fred Hammond's "Let the Praise Begin."

Are you ready for your blessing? Are you ready?
Are you ready for your miracle?

I was.

The surgery was supposed to last eight hours, but it took only three. Something had changed in the days between the MRI and the surgery. The doctors said that my spine had made an unexpected rapid recovery.

I smiled at this news, but was by no means surprised by it. I believe God miraculously healed me before the surgeon's scalpel ever touched me. I had faith that I was healed and was ready to leave the hospital.

After a grueling rehab, I made it back in four weeks to start the final preseason game at linebacker against the Green Bay Packers at historic Lambeau Field. Months earlier, they said there was a chance I wouldn't play another down in the NFL. But here I was, suiting up, ready for action.

I didn't miss a single regular season game that year.

Throughout the whole process, I never doubted God, and He showed Himself strong! This life lesson taught me that believing is seeing. It is often said, *I will believe it when I see it.* That is not what brings the desired result. We must believe and see the desired results in our spirits before we can see them in reality.

11.

BALTIMORE BOUND

Whatever you do, you need courage.

—Ralph Waldo Emerson

DURING the 1999 campaign, I suffered elbow and ankle injuries, too. The pain was intense, but I wanted to be on the field for my teammates on Sundays. I didn't want to let them down. I was also motivated by the long road I took to the NFL. I knew how hard it was to finally get on the field and that there was always going to be someone else who'd gladly take my spot on the roster if I missed a game. I'd seen that story line play out time and time again over the course of my career, and I wasn't about to see it happen to me. I was the special teams captain and I was going to lead by example. I did just about everything in my power to ensure that I suited up on Sundays. Come one p.m., I was always ready to go. Coach Johnson used to say, "You can't make the club from the tub!" He was right.

Many of my teammates knew about my injuries and told me that I inspired *them* by fighting through the pain each week. If seeing me take the field—with my elbow, back, and ankles wrapped up in what must have looked like miles of athletic tape—helped motivate the Miami Dolphins, then I was going to do everything in my power to take the field.

I appeared in all sixteen regular-season games in 1999 and played in both of our play-off contests that season. Though our 62–7 loss to the Jaguars in the divisional round of the NFL play-offs made for a fourth straight unfortunate end to the season, I was humbled to learn that the Dolphins named me their recipient of the Ed Block Courage Award that March.

The Ed Block Courage Award Foundation is dedicated to improving the lives of abused, neglected, and at-risk children. Each year, the foundation recognizes one player from each team as its recipients of the award. They're often the individuals who triumphed in the face of adversity. My being chosen to represent the '99 Dolphins meant that my teammates recognized the physical pain I went through on a weekly basis that season, and respected the mental toughness it took for me to take the field each week.

Chanda and I made the trip back to Baltimore, our former home, for the two-day awards ceremony. While in Charm City for the event, we revisited all of our old haunts and met up with some old friends from the Stallions days. It felt great to be back in Baltimore, a city we both loved so much.

At the ceremony, I was introduced to Ozzie Newsome, the general manager of the Baltimore Ravens. The Ravens were the NFL team that essentially spelled the end of the Stallions. They'd been in Baltimore for four seasons, but had yet to field a play-off team. The city's fans, as I had no doubt they would, rallied around the franchise and made it their own. People in Baltimore were as crazy about the struggling Ravens as they were about the much more successful Orioles. Football was in Baltimore's blood, and the city was glad to have the NFL game back in its grasp.

I'd grown up rooting *against* Ozzie Newsome when he was a Hall of Fame tight end on the Cleveland Browns who always seemed to give my Houston Oilers fits. Now he was running the NFL franchise in Baltimore. My contract was up with the Dolphins and I was back where I was four years earlier, wondering about my NFL future. I'd put together a very productive four seasons in Miami, but my recent string of surgeries seemed to scare off some teams.

Ozzie and I had a very good conversation. Like me, Ozzie wasn't a man of many words and was by no means a rah-rah type. He went about his business by working hard and leading by example. We saw eye to eye on a lot of things, and our approaches to life and football were essentially the same. It wouldn't always be easy, but doing things the *right way* would always work out best in the end.

I left the Ed Block Courage Award dinner that night with a really positive feeling about a potential homecoming in Baltimore. When I left the city for Miami four years earlier, I was a champion with thirteen straight wins under my belt. Perhaps it was time to come back and be a champion in Baltimore once again?

Meanwhile, in Miami, things were definitely changing. After the 62–7 loss to the Jaguars in the play-offs, Dan Marino, the franchise's starting quarterback for the past seventeen seasons, retired. Jimmy Johnson, despite three straight trips to the play-offs, stepped away from the game, too. Much of the roster would look different in 2000, and I hadn't heard from the team's front office about extending my contract.

Though I felt good about my conversation with Ozzie Newsome, months went by and I hadn't heard from the Ravens, Dolphins, or any of the NFL's twenty-nine other teams. I spent the off-season training at Cris Carter's speed camp in Boca Raton, Florida. Cris's work ethic was tremendous, and I saw firsthand why he is a Pro Football Hall of Famer. I prepared myself for the next assignment, confident that a call would come. I was in great physical shape and I was mentally ready for the challenge. I just needed a chance.

We were having a cookout with some friends when the phone call I'd been waiting for all summer came.

During my morning reading, the following verses from 1 Kings 17:2–6 spoke to my spirit:

"Then the word of the Lord came to Elijah: 'Leave here, turn eastward and hide in the Kerith Ravine, east of the Jordan. You will drink from the brook, and I have directed the ravens to supply you with food there.' So he did what the Lord had told him. He went to the Kerith Ravine, east of the Jordan, and stayed there. The ravens brought him bread and meat in the morning and bread and meat in the evening, and he drank from the brook."

The call that day came from George Kokinis of the Baltimore Ravens. Unbelievable!

George said they would like to fly me to Baltimore for a workout. I caught a flight up and worked out for Jack Del Rio, Baltimore's linebackers coach, and Marvin Lewis, the team's defensive coordinator. The workout went well and the Ravens signed me to a free-agent contract. Thank you, Jesus! I was going back to Baltimore.

The Ravens will feed you!

I got to Baltimore and was amazed by the good fortune I'd stepped into. There were four future Pro Football Hall of Famers on the Ravens roster, with big Jonathan Ogden at left tackle, two-time Super Bowl champion Shannon Sharpe at tight end, All-World defensive back Rod Woodson at safety, and arguably the best player in the entire sport, Ray Lewis, at linebacker.

I'd been on good teams before and suited up with Dan Marino for four years in Miami, but I'd never been on a team as rich with talent as this one. Brian Billick was the head coach, and he was quite a bit different from Coach Johnson. Unlike in Miami, where the summers were downright brutal, Coach Billick wanted to ensure we were fresh for the regular season. Training camp was by no means easy, but it wasn't anything like the six-week grind that we endured each year in South Florida.

Coach Billick knew he had a team made of veterans and treated us as such. There were no curfews or bed checks. He expected us to be accountable and act like responsible adults. The "rules" were more or less unspoken: Show up and come ready to play. He treated us like men, and in turn, we all wanted to perform to the best of our abilities for him.

Coach Billick's staff was one of the best ever assembled. Linebackers coach Jack Del Rio and I immediately hit it off, as we both had great respect for each other's careers as players. Our defensive coordinator, Marvin Lewis, had an eye for talent and could draw up a defensive scheme with the very best of them. Rex Ryan, the current head coach of the New York Jets, was in charge of our defensive line. Mike Smith, a wonderful man who now coaches the Atlanta Falcons, was a defensive assistant on that team, too. The amount of knowledge and experience on that coaching staff couldn't be quantified.

Our team was unified through several external factors. The Ravens still had never made the play-offs, and that shared desire fueled us. The city of Baltimore hadn't seen a champion since our Stallions team left for Montreal in 1995. There was that, too. But the central motivating force behind the 2000 Baltimore Ravens was Ray Lewis.

Following a 1999 regular season in which he led the league

in tackles, Ray headed down to Atlanta to attend a Super Bowl party. Sometime after midnight, a fight broke out in the street outside the nightclub where the party was being held. Two men were stabbed and killed.

Ray was arrested the following morning in front of his three sons. He, along with two others, was indicted on murder and aggravated-assault charges. His first night in prison, Ray heard a whisper in his ear.

"Can you hear me now?"

God had never spoken to him so clearly. In his prison cell that evening, Ray became a different man. He'd never be the same again.

Ray was absolved of the charges, pleading guilty to obstruction of justice in exchange for testimony against his codefendants. Those two young men were acquitted of the charges in June.

It was the biggest story that entire NFL off-season, and all anyone wanted to talk about when we arrived at training camp in July. Coach Billick knew that the incident could either tear our team apart and serve as a distraction or galvanize us and bring us closer. It did the latter.

We rallied around Ray and we rallied around one another. After every practice that summer, reporters pressed Ray with questions about the case. The media was nothing compared to the opposing teams' fans. At road games, Ray heard everything you could possibly imagine. They'd call him a murderer and they'd shout racist epithets from their seats. What the opposing crowds didn't realize was that those words—and those awful, hateful names—didn't faze Ray Lewis or cause him to crumble. They motivated him.

Those angry words put him into a gladiator state of mind. He'd use the vitriol from the opposing fans as fuel for his inner fire. We'd rally around it, too.

"If they're that bold to put my reputation on the line, then I'm as bold as they are to fight for it," he'd say.

Ray was willing to do whatever was necessary to defend his good name. We watched him fight; his spirit was contagious and spread throughout the entire Ravens locker room. We truly had an "us against the world" mentality that season.

Though he was just twenty-five years old and surrounded by veterans who'd been in the league for several more years than he had, Ray was our leader. We fed off his desire to be the best who ever played. We fed off his desire to defend his honor.

On the field, he was the single best player in the league. Off of it, he was a man evolving into a new phase of his life. I saw Ray's relationship with God transform during that trying period. He was a regular in our Bible-study group in Baltimore, and he and I would often sit together for long hours after practice, going through various passages.

We became more than merely close friends. We became brothers.

He dubbed me "Juice," saying that I was "always refreshing." I'd call him "Ray Lew" or "Sugar." Sometimes I'd describe myself as a gazelle. Ray would shake his head and explain that lions—him, in this case—usually got the best of the gazelles. The linebackers room was where we'd put long hours of work in, but it was also a place where jokes would be cracked and stunts would be pulled. Every day, it was something different. And every day, someone else—whether it was Ray, Jamie Sharper, Peter Boulware, Cornell Brown, Brad Jackson, or myself—was catching the brunt of it.

Ray and I connected on a spiritual level, too. He told me that through me, he saw God's work. He saw with his own two eyes that you didn't need to be the biggest or fastest or strongest physical specimen to succeed. As long as you had your mind, your heart, and the will to fight, you could accomplish great feats.

Those were difficult times for Ray, and I wanted him to know that no matter what he was going through, I'd always be there for him. We never focused on the strife, but instead looked toward the future. We spoke about brighter days on the horizon.

I had hundreds of one-on-one conversations with Ray Lewis over the course of that 2000 season. He'd thank me for being a source of joy during such a tumultuous time. Little did I know back then that in the coming years, he'd grow to become an important rock in *my* life. He'd serve as a source of light and great comfort during some of my darkest hours.

I had a feeling the 2000 Ravens were a special group of men as early as the preseason. Though the games don't technically count in the standings, we went 4–0 in our exhibition games. Our defense jelled, and the positivity oozing from Coach Billick was contagious. I played primarily on the special teams unit, teaming up with Robert Bailey and Billy Davis, serving as the team's tackle. I chased down punt and kick returners with everything I had, doing my best to pin our opponents back as far into their own territory as I possibly could.

From there, the defense did the job. And, man, what a defense we had.

We won four of our first five regular season games, shutting three of our first four opponents out. Even during a three-game losing streak in the middle of the season, our defense gave up only ten, fourteen, and nine points, respectively, in the defeats. Led by Ray in the middle, we didn't give up a single hundred-yard rusher the entire regular season. We surrendered the least points ever for a team playing a sixteen-game schedule. By most accounts, the 2000 Ravens fielded the greatest defense the NFL has ever seen.

In week nine, Coach Billick made a controversial coaching decision when he replaced our starting quarterback, Tony Banks, with our backup, Trent Dilfer. The offense had been struggling, and Coach Billick thought it was time for a shake-up. Trent was a former first-round pick of the Tampa Bay Buccaneers, but had experienced many ups and downs during his time there. In the spring of 2000, he signed with Baltimore, still confident he could be an effective NFL signal caller. Many of us could relate to Trent's story. We were sort of like the island of misfit toys in Baltimore: a bunch of guys discarded by other teams along the way, motivated by other people's doubts. I always admired Trent's confidence in himself and his abilities. He knew he might have to wait awhile before being given the opportunity to shine, but once he got one, he wouldn't squander it.

In Trent's first game as the starter, we lost 9–6 to the Steelers. He didn't play as well as he wanted to, and assured the team that week in practice that he'd be far better the following week versus the Bengals. We traveled to Cincinnati as losers of three straight games, with the season more or less on the line.

After a slow start, Trent caught fire. We beat the Bengals 27–7, then took down the defending AFC Champion Tennessee Titans in Nashville the following week. We shut out the Dallas Cowboys in week twelve and beat the Cleveland Browns and San Diego Chargers in back-to-back blowout victories. We were red-hot. Winners of five straight games, we headed into a battle with the Arizona Cardinals focused on a single goal—bringing the Lombardi Trophy back to the city of Baltimore.

That was when tragedy stopped us in our tracks.

Jermaine Lewis was our kick and punt return man and the spark plug of our special teams group. He showed up every day to practice with a smile on his face, excited to get on the field and make a play. Only five-foot-seven, he had the heart of a champion and an unbelievable drive within him.

On the Tuesday before our West Coast trip to the Arizona desert, Jermaine and his eight-and-a-half-month pregnant wife,

Imara, went for their weekly checkup with their obstetrician. They were told that their child's heart had ceased beating. He was stillborn at eight months.

The news quickly spread around the locker room the next morning and we were all distraught. Jermaine was a brother of ours, and we knew how eager both he and Imara were for the arrival of their new son, Geronimo.

Though he was still grieving, Jermaine wanted to join the team and play against the Cardinals that Sunday afternoon. Coach Billick wouldn't let him, insisting that he would regret for the rest of his life leaving his wife when she needed him most. A pastor visited Jermaine and Imara that week, staying long hours at their home as they coped with the news. I reached out to Jermaine and shared my deepest condolences. I couldn't have possibly imagined his pain.

We rallied around him and won an emotional game on the road that weekend.

The following week, Jermaine was ready to play. It was our season finale and we were up against the 9–6 New York Jets. A win would give us seven straight victories heading into the play-offs and would eliminate New York from postseason contention.

Ray and I spoke to Jermaine before the game and saw a determined look in his eyes. I thought back to the 601-yard, four-touchdown performance Danny Barrett had had following the death of his brother. Tragedy can shatter a man's will. It can also inspire and lift us to new heights.

Ray led us in a team prayer before kickoff and we dedicated the forthcoming effort to Geronimo.

Jermaine Lewis went out and had the single greatest game of his NFL career that day. He tied an NFL record by returning two punts for touchdowns, one for fifty-four yards and the other for eighty-nine. Chris McAlister, our star cornerback, returned an interception ninety-eight yards for a score. We toppled the Jets 34–20 and headed into the play-offs as one of the hottest teams in the league.

After the emotional win, Jermaine was handed the game ball by Coach Billick. He broke down in tears. There wasn't a dry eye in that locker room that afternoon. "I really just tried to stay focused," Jermaine told reporters afterward. "I really don't know how I did it, but I know the Lord helped me through it."

God works in amazing ways. He wasn't finished.

We won our first-ever play-off game as a franchise over the Broncos in the wild-card round, and upset the Tennessee Titans a week later. We traveled out to Oakland as big underdogs to face the Raiders in the AFC Championship Game.

In the locker room before kickoff, Shannon Sharpe asked Ray Lewis how many points the defense needed from the offense to ensure a win. "Give us ten, Shannon. All we need is ten. If you can score ten, we'll take care of the rest," Ray said.

Sure enough, Shannon took a pass from Trent ninety-six yards for a touchdown in the first half. Our kicker, Matt Stover, would add three field goals. The defense had their ten points and six more. As Ray promised, they took care of the rest. Tony Siragusa got to their quarterback Rich Gannon early on, and the rest of the guys shut down their high-flying offense over the course of the next four quarters. It was by no means pretty, but that's just how we liked it.

We won 16–3.

Ten points was really all we needed.

By God's grace, we were headed to the Super Bowl.

12.

SUPER SUNDAYS

I learned this, at least, by my experiment: that if one advances confidently in the direction of his dreams, and endeavors to live the life which he has imagined, he will meet with a success unexpected in common hours.

—Henry David Thoreau

WE arrived in Tampa Bay, the host city for Super Bowl XXXV, with a clear objective in mind: We wanted to leave the city seven days later as world champions. We wouldn't accept anything less.

The New York Giants were our opponents, and they, like us, were coming off an impressive victory in their championship game. We studied New York's game tapes and prepared for a battle with the NFC's best team.

We quickly realized, however, that the week wouldn't just be about the Ravens and Giants. Everywhere we went, the conversation was focused on Ray and the incident in Atlanta. The New York media contingent was ready to dive deep into the night that Ray was ready to put behind him. At every mandatory event, especially during Super Bowl Media Day, Ray was asked questions about Atlanta.

In the hours after Media Day, there was incredible tension in our locker room. Ray had just been grilled by hundreds of reporters for an hour straight. It was quiet, a rarity for our team. Tony Siragusa, Shannon Sharpe, and Ray were all known for their locker room chatter and hijinks. But you could hear a pin drop that afternoon.

Qadry knew what had to be done. He put on some hip-hop music, whatever song was popular at the time, and started dancing. We all lightened up and shook our heads in disbelief. Then Brad Jackson, one of our linebackers, got up and broke out his best Ray Lewis impression. Art Modell, the team's owner, had given all of us handheld video cameras earlier in the week. With the music blaring and the rest of the team rolling in laughter, Brad did Ray's signature "squirrel dance" in the middle of the room. We all pressed RECORD on our handhelds and captured the routine.

One by one, the guys got up and imitated Ray's dance. Each one was better than the last.

Then Qadry pointed at me. "It's your turn, Juice!"

I shook my head. "No, no, no. I don't dance. You know that, man." I could chase a kick returner down and offer a few good words of inspiration, but *dancing* was not something I was known for.

Then the whole team started to pile on. They wanted me to break out my moves.

Soon, fifty-three men were chanting, "Juice! Juice! Juice!"

I looked around the room. These were my brothers. I took a second to collect myself and thought, *Ah, why not?*

I got up, with Ray Lewis sitting right next to me, and calmly walked to the center of a giant circle of clapping and dancing teammates. When the beat dropped, so did I, right to the ground. I broke out my very best "squirrel dance" routine, nailing it. The room erupted with cheers. Ray might have been laughing the hardest.

"Juiiiiiiiiice!" he shouted.

It was a stressful afternoon, and of all the things in the world, my dance moves helped lighten the mood. To this day, Qadry and Ray remind me of that moment. Ray claims there's video footage of it somewhere. I tell him I have no interest in seeing it!

We had a solid week of practice, and Coach Billick brought in guest speakers like Hank Aaron and Smokin' Joe Frazier to lend some perspective. We knew this was our time.

Personally, during my reading time, the spirit impressed on my heart the Israelites at the battle of Jericho. The story goes as follows:

1. Now Jericho [a fenced town with high walls] was tightly closed because of the Israelites; no one went out or came in.
2. And the Lord said to Joshua, See, I have given Jericho, its king and mighty men of valor, into your hands.
3. You shall march around the enclosure, all the men of war going around the city once. This you shall do for six days.
4. And seven priests shall bear before the ark seven trumpets of rams' horns; and on the seventh day you

shall march around the enclosure seven times, and the priests shall blow the trumpets.

5. When they make a long blast with the ram's horn and you hear the sound of the trumpet, all the people shall shout with a great shout; and the wall of the enclosure shall fall down in its place and the people shall go up [over it], every man straight before him.

Tampa Bay's Raymond James Stadium was our Jericho. Every evening that week, I drove around the stadium just one time, praying that God would be glorified through us. On Super Bowl Sunday, I came out on the field early and circled it seven times, praying God would use us in a special way.

By kickoff, there were no more distractions, no more nasty headlines, no more external forces to worry about. It was time to play some football.

My parents and Chanda were in the crowd, and I'd arranged for tickets for my best friends from high school, Todd and Karl. My sister, Myla, made the trip to Florida, but opted to watch the game from her hotel room. That was Myla—always supporting me, just not a big fan of football!

We lost the coin toss and the Giants elected to receive. I lined up with Billy Davis and we gave each other the look we'd given each other before opening kickoffs all season long. One of us was going to start this game off right. Ray pulled me aside and said, "Ain't nobody going to beat you to the football, Juice. *Nobody.*"

Our placekicker, Matt Stover, booted the ball off deep to New York's return man, Ron Dixon. I shed one blocker, then two, and zeroed in on the number 86 across Dixon's chest. I dived at his waist, grabbed him around the hips, and tossed him to the ground. I'd just made the first tackle of the Super Bowl!

I was so fired up that I jumped to my feet, crouched, and did a little Billy "White Shoes" Johnson celebratory dance. I ran to the sideline and high-fived Ray.

Trent tossed a perfect thirty-eight-yard touchdown pass to Brandon Stokley, and we took an early 7–0 lead in the first quarter. I knew that was all the defense really needed.

As we lined up for a second-half kickoff, up by ten points, I gave a look to Jermaine, standing a few yards behind me in our end zone. I had a good feeling he'd make his mark. He caught the ball, made a cutback, and was gone. Eighty-four yards. Touchdown!

I'll never forget the image of Jermaine celebrating that score in the Super Bowl, on the biggest of stages. After all he'd been through in the past month, he had a smile as wide as could be on his face. We all knew that one was for Geronimo.

We won Super Bowl XXXV by a score of 34–7. As I did with the Grey Cup so many years ago, I took the Lombardi Trophy with both of my hands and kissed it. Players, my ex-teammate Dan Marino for one, go their entire careers without getting the opportunity to hoist the Lombardi. Here I was, with my family and best friends in the crowd, clutching it close to my chest.

Ray Lewis won the game's MVP award and cried tears of joy in the locker room. Trent played wonderfully, proving he was a first-rate quarterback after all. I had my best game as a Raven, making five special teams tackles, including the first one of the evening. With the Super Bowl victory that night, I became the first and only player in football history to win a Grey Cup and a Super Bowl for teams in the same city. I'd forever be a part of Baltimore sports history. Or, at the very least, the answer to a pretty cool trivia question.

———

AFTER the victory parade through downtown Baltimore the following week, the 2001 off-season began. I was a free agent yet again. Though I loved being a Raven and wanted nothing more than to defend our title the next year, the team did not offer me a contract extension.

My assignment was over.

I used to really struggle moving from team to team. Human nature yearns for stability, but if not kept in perspective, comfort can easily become complacency. We are called to grow in life.

I learned that every assignment lasts for only a season; then it is time to move on to the next one. My next assignment was with the St. Louis Rams. I went to training camp and ended up getting cut for the first time in my career. This was uncharted territory for me, because I always got the job in the past. I had already found an apartment and assumed I would be on the team come the start of the regular season.

But it wasn't in God's plan. There is no better fertilizer in life than adversity, and it was growing season. The Rams' head coach, Mike Martz, said they were releasing me because they had some injuries on the defensive line and needed to bring in another player. I had always been on the bubble throughout my career, but always found a way to overcome.

All I could do was just go back to the apartment and sleep. Chanda was still living in our home in Baltimore, so it was just me and God in the apartment those nights. I found a local gym to work out in, and on Tuesday, September 11, I witnessed one of our nation's greatest tragedies unfold on TV, while running on the treadmill.

I was stunned by the horrific loss of life. Being released, while personally devastating, paled in comparison to what was happening in New York. That following Friday, I was watching the memorial service on television when revelation came through the words of President Bush.

Addressing the hundreds in attendance and millions around the world, he gave a remarkable speech. And in just five words, he stoked the fire of resilience within me.

"Adversity introduces us to ourselves," he said.

Adversity introduces us to ourselves.

Through adversity, one is able to take a reflective look at your character and resiliency! Those words shook me from my complacency and renewed my desire to get back to work. I returned back home to Maryland to await my opportunity. No calls came, and I started thinking about my transition plan from the game.

Finally, in week eight of the 2001 NFL season, the Rams called because one of their linebackers broke his wrist and a roster spot had opened up. I was headed back to St. Louis!

When I got there, I immediately hit it off with a man whose NFL journey was as unorthodox as—if not more than—mine. Kurt Warner, the team's star quarterback and the MVP of the 1999 NFL season, took the scenic route to the league, too. After going undrafted out of Northern Iowa, Kurt was released by the Green Bay Packers during training camp in 1994. Forced to put his NFL plans on hold when he, too, spent nights looking at a phone that never rang, Kurt worked at a Hy-Vee grocery store in Cedar Falls, Iowa, stocking shelves for $5.50 an hour. Times were tough, but he wouldn't let his NFL dream die.

Offered a tryout while he was still working the night shift at the Hy-Vee, Kurt tried out for the Arena Football League's Iowa Barnstormers and made the team. He spent the next three years in the Arena League before getting his shot with the Amsterdam Admirals of NFL Europe. After a season serving as Jake Delhomme's backup overseas, he finally made it to the NFL in 1998 with the Rams as their third-string quarterback. His opportunity came after the team's starting quarterback, Trent Green, went down with an injury during the 1999 preseason.

Though others around the league had never heard of him, and even the team's own fan base had its doubts, Kurt got his chance. He knew that was all he ever needed. He took the Rams right to the Super Bowl, leading the franchise to its first Lombardi Trophy.

Now, led by Kurt on offense and All-Pro defensive back Aeneas Williams on defense, we went 14–2 during the regular season and steamrolled through the play-offs to the Super Bowl. Few players get the opportunity to play in one Super Bowl. Here I was, playing in my second in consecutive years. I was blessed.

Up against the New England Patriots, we were heavily favored, having had the better regular season record and the league's most feared offense. The entire Brigance family and my mother-in-law drove to New Orleans from Houston, so we were well represented.

Driving to the stadium that night was somewhat surreal because of such a heavy military presence in light of the 9/11 attacks. We had to go through checkpoints after just about every two hundred feet. Once we got to the Superdome, I made my way to midfield to greet a familiar face.

"Take it all in, Izz. Savor this moment," I said as I put my arm around my former teammate and fellow Rice Owl Larry Izzo.

After five great years with the Dolphins, Larry had signed a free-agent contract with the Patriots the previous March. Brothers-in-arms for four seasons in Miami on Mike Westhoff's special teams unit, we were now going head-to-head with a Lombardi Trophy on the line. My one job for the evening was to block Larry Izzo. Larry's one job for the evening was to block O. J. Brigance. It had to be the first time two Rice Owls squared off in a Super Bowl, and we were both thrilled to represent Owl Nation on the grandest of stages.

The mood of the game was unique from the start. When it

came time for the pregame introductions, we were introduced first with our offensive starters. Torry Holt, Isaac Bruce, Marshall Faulk, and Kurt were all greeted with cheers as they came out of the tunnel.

When it was time for the Patriots to be introduced, though, they did something that had never been done in Super Bowl history. They chose to be introduced as a team and the stadium erupted. They showed a united front from the beginning that would emulate the strength the American people were feeling.

The game was a tug-of-war for three and a half quarters. Our defense stopped the Patriots on a key fourth-quarter drive, and their punter booted the ball deep into our territory. Dré Bly, our return man, received the punt and dashed for a twenty-five-yard gain. My assignment on the play was to block none other than number 53, Larry Izzo.

Going up against each other for the first time in our careers, I blocked Larry and opened up a hole for Dré. To this day, I stand behind the fact that the play was completely legal! Larry went flying to the ground, however, acting as though he were being held. He deserved an Oscar for the performance. What a thespian. Sure enough, the official threw a yellow flag. Penalty!

Larry got the best of me on that one, but years later, he admitted that I didn't hold him on the play. Coach Johnson was right all those years back at training camp. Larry *would* do whatever was necessary to win. I saw it firsthand in Super Bowl XXXVI.

The game was tied at 17 with 1:30 left in regulation. The Patriots got the ball with no time-outs remaining. I knew in my heart that if we could just get to overtime, we would win the game. But we wouldn't get that chance. Tom Brady led his team downfield on a game-winning drive, and kicker Adam Vinatieri nailed a forty-eight-yard field goal attempt as time expired.

The Patriots were Super Bowl champions. Their sideline

erupted and ran across the field in jubilant celebration, as our sideline was cast into utter disbelief and despair. Our 14–2 record might just as well have been 2–14. We lost the one that counted. Red, white, and blue confetti rained from the sky to the tune "We Are the Champions." Security quickly roped off the field, pushing us aside as if we didn't have tickets to the game. We retreated to our locker room, dejected. I tried to put on a brave front, but this one hurt.

The next off-season, I was once again a free agent looking for an opportunity. Training camps started in July, and a couple of weeks in, I got a call from Scott Pioli, now the Patriots general manager, inviting me to come up for a workout. My last tryout for Pioli was when he was with the Browns in 1995. This one went a lot better than that one, and I was offered a contract on the spot. I signed it and looked forward to the chance to play for the great Bill Belichick.

Another perk? I'd be reunited with my man "Izz"!

During one of my first practices, I was running side by side with Larry down the field when I felt a sharp pain in my back that forced me to pull up. The trainers came out and escorted me inside to check me out. I ended up getting an MRI and they determined it was back spasms. My back locked up and I was bedridden for a couple of days. This sealed my fate, because, as Jimmy Johnson used to say, "You can't make the club from the tub!"

The Patriots released me, but Pioli said they would bring me back once I got healthy. A man of his word, they did re-sign me. But it was just for one game. After a 44–7 win over the New York Jets, the Patriots let me go once again. I caught on with the Rams for the remainder of the season, but missed out on any more Super Bowl appearances. We finished 7–9, marking the end of the Rams' "Greatest Show on Turf" era, and my time as an NFL player.

I was thirty-two years old and was in a good place mentally with my life and football career. I had nothing more to achieve on the gridiron, no more naysayers to prove wrong. It's rare that a player gets to determine when his playing days are over.

I knew that it was my time.

13.

NOW WHAT?

Take delight in the Lord, and he will give you the desires of your heart.

—Psalms 37:4

MY entire life, I wanted to be an NFL football player. I achieved
that dream, won a Super Bowl, played in another, and was recognized as the NFLPA's Unsung Hero in 1999. I'd done everything I could have ever imagined as a football player in my seven
seasons in the NFL.

But now I was thirty-two years old and out of work.

Postretirement is an incredibly vexing time for most NFL
players. For years, you're a part of a team, striving for a unified goal, and getting paid to do what you love. But the average NFL career lasts roughly three years, and even the best
players in the game are rarely still active at thirty-five. Whereas
the rest of the American workforce is just hitting its stride in

its mid-thirties, an NFL player's career is usually over by then.

So, what do you do when the crowds go silent? It's a question most ex-players struggle with immensely.

Chanda and I had a difficult time figuring the answer out ourselves. For as much as I loved being a part of the NFL world, Chanda did, too. She made friends with the other players' wives, hosted events, and became a vital part of the community no matter which city we were in. Chanda was as much of a presence during our NFL days as I was.

Now, for the first time since I was an eight-year-old boy, I didn't know what I wanted to do with my life. Chanda and I prayed about our future, wide-open but daunting. Fortunately, I was wise with my finances as a player, both in Canada and the U.S., and we had some money saved.

"You've achieved everything you've ever put your mind to, O.J. What do you *want* to do?" Chanda asked me one day.

I knew I wanted to make a difference in some way. I knew I wanted to follow God's lead and live life in a righteous manner. I knew I still wanted to be part of a team—not necessarily a football one, per se—but some team.

After several months of deep thought and prayer, God dropped into my spirit one night and suggested I meet with Coach Billick. On top of being a wonderful head coach, Coach Billick was a mentor of mine. He'd followed my career and kept in touch with Chanda and me even after I left the Ravens. I wanted some help with my résumé and also, if he was willing, planned on asking him for a letter of recommendation that I could share with potential employers. I'd done internships in broadcasting and marketing, but I thought I might want to try my hand at coaching.

When I called Coach Billick to set up a meeting, he asked me several questions that I hadn't yet asked myself. Where did I want to be in five years? Ten years? What kind of difference did I want to make?

He then asked me whether I wanted to re-join the Ravens.

I was thrown off. "What do mean, *re-join* the Ravens?" I asked.

As it turned out, Earnest Byner, the team's director of player programs, was leaving his position with the Ravens to pursue *his* dream of being an NFL coach. As of that week, there was a job available in the Ravens' front office. Coach Billick was unaware that Chanda and I were living right down the road at the time and believed it wasn't merely some happy coincidence that I'd called him that day. It was more. I was there for a reason.

What *was* the job, exactly? Well, that was the intriguing part. Coach Billick said it was loosely defined at the time and that I would be able to mold and shape the position into whatever I wanted it to be. The main focus of the job was helping the players with everything in their lives off the field. From financial advice to relationship guidance to aiding rookies in getting settled with a home in Baltimore—the director of player programs was the individual players could turn to for tutelage in all things nonfootball.

When I met with Coach Billick in person a few days later, we discussed the position in greater detail. Ozzie Newsome said that before the Ravens offered me the job formally, they wanted to see what I envisioned for the director of player programs role. Ozzie asked that I prepare a formal proposal and present it to the two of them.

I got home and shared the details of my day with Chanda and we prayed on it. This whole transition process had been tough for her to accept, because she initially thought I was giving up due to being released. Far from it. When your passion is gone, it is time to move on.

During my time of reflection, I realized the position would

be right for me. After all, it was what I had been doing unoffi-
cially for years. Excited about the opportunity, I met with our
team chaplain, Rod Hairston, to get insight on the transitional
phases of a professional athlete. Rod is a great man of God and
a treasure trove of wisdom. After meeting with him, I had the
vision. Every aspect of my playing career would give me experiential knowledge to help influence the lives of my men. I prepared my proposal for Ozzie, centered around the four tenets of
player development:

1. Continuing education
2. Financial education
3. Internships
4. Players Assistance Program (PAP)

Ozzie liked my proposal, and the Ravens offered me the position when I met with them the following week. But I didn't
accept the job right away. I needed Chanda to be on board.

As part of my new position, she would be asked to join the
team in an organizational role, too. She had always been such an
important part of my life as a player, but there was rarely someone she could go to with questions within the various organizations I played for. A good man is only as good as the woman by
his side. Ozzie and Coach Billick asked Chanda to work with
and serve as a mentor for all of the Ravens players' and coaches'
wives. She loved the idea of working in such a capacity, but I
wanted to ensure that this was really what we wanted to do in
the next phase of our lives.

We prayed about it for several nights. After about a week,
Ozzie said he needed an answer. He was headed to the NFL
draft Scouting Combine and had to fill both positions. After several more discussions and prayers, Chanda and I agreed that this
was something we wanted to pursue. God had presented this

opportunity for a reason, and now it was our time to give back to the game by sharing our years of experience and knowledge.

I was eager to share what I had learned throughout my career to help the men succeed. One of my passions is motivating people to take advantage of their opportunities.

I thought back to my days at Rice, when I served as the student career adviser. I loved that role. With the Ravens, I could do so much more. I'd seen it all in my years as a player. There were good things—players going back to school in their off-seasons to graduate or earn master's degrees, community service activities, to name a few. But there was also a lot of bad—guys blowing entire paychecks on unnecessary expenses, family members coming out of the woodwork with their palms outstretched, looking for handouts. I knew that I could make a difference not only with rookies, but with veterans. I could serve as their eyes and ears, their guiding hand.

I started in March of 2004, and during my first few weeks on the job, I reached out to several veteran directors of player programs around the league and discovered many passionate, like-minded men and women who were heavily invested in the well-being of their players. The NFL was just beginning to take a more proactive approach to assisting players with their transition into, during, and out of the game. I knew I could be a leader in this area of focus.

I implemented several new programs and launched new initiatives. I brought in different speakers on each topic to offer their insight. For a conversation on how to be a professional, I tapped into the expertise of the Ravens' team owner, Steve Bisciotti. The young guys hung on to his every word. He would say things like, "You can live like a king for a day or a prince for the rest of your life." Mr. Bisciotti would emphasize that if you focused all of your time and energy on your craft, you would come out much farther ahead than if you tried to be a part-time entrepreneur in a "get-rich-quick" scheme. He spoke from the heart, because he, too, wanted the men to be successful in their lives both on the field and off.

The chance to glean wisdom from veterans like Ed Reed, Derrick Mason, and Ray Lewis was priceless to them, too. Those guys were icons to the younger players, and having them take the time to offer their personal experiences, both good and bad, was always so greatly appreciated.

Ozzie would speak to the men as well. He'd also guide me. When I was selected to serve on a league committee, I asked Ozzie for some advice. He dropped a nugget on me that serves me well to this day: "You must know the people in the room and their end intentions."

I affectionately referred to my first Ravens draft class as my "firstborn." The opportunity to impart wisdom into these men was a great privilege for me. Dwan Edwards, Devard Darling, Roderick Green, Josh Harris, Clarence Moore, Derek Abney and Brian Rimpf. These men helped me to grow as they grew. I would often remind them that they were CEOs of their own major corporations. Every decision they would make—good or bad—would affect their companies' bottom lines. I fed them the statistics over and over again—the average NFL career lasts only a little more than three years. I'd tell them, "Take advantage of the opportunity you have now and it could be a financial springboard for the rest of your life."

I encouraged them to be champions both on and off the field. The NFL measures this title by wins and losses. While I was in Miami, God revealed to me that it was so much more.

There are eight attributes of a true C. H. A. M. P. I. O. N.
Commit.

A champion must commit everything to Jesus, mind, body, and spirit.

Proverbs 16:3 says, "Commit to the Lord whatever you do

and your plans will succeed." There is no success without commitment, and no lasting success without commitment to Christ.

Heart.

A champion has a pure heart. Proverbs 4:23 says, "Above all else, guard your heart, for it is the wellspring of life." If you allow garbage into your heart, garbage will come back out.

Attitude.

A champion has the right attitude. According to Christian author and pastor Chuck Swindoll, life is ten percent what happens to you and ninety percent how you react to it. We rarely have control over what happens to us, but we always have control over how we choose to react to it.

Morals.

A champion has morals. You can't live and treat people any kind of way and expect good things to come back to you. The Bible says, "Do not be deceived; God will not be mocked. As a man sows, so shall he reap."

Perseverance.

Champions have great perseverance. There will always be trials and tests in life. There is no trial that comes upon us that God hasn't prepared us for.

Initiative.

A champion takes the initiative, even and especially when opportunities require a leap of faith on our part. Matthew 7:7 says, "Ask and you will receive; seek and you will find; knock and the door will be opened to you." The world says, "Show me and I will believe you," while God says, "Believe me and I will show you."

Opportunity.

Champions make the most of every opportunity. Ephesians 5:16 talks about this. We are owed nothing in this world, but by God's grace we will get opportunities to do extraordinary things. What we do with those opportunities is up to us.

Never underestimate the power of God!

A champion never underestimates the power of God to do the impossible. First Corinthians 2:9 declares, "'What no eye has seen, what no ear has heard, and what no human mind has conceived'—the things God has prepared for those who love him." We should never let man's limitations restrict God's possibilities. We are all uniquely and wonderfully made by God to do extraordinary things.

14.

THE RAVENS WAY

From everyone who has been given much, much will be demanded; and from the one who has been entrusted with much, much more will be asked.

—Luke 12:48

RAY Lewis was still the heart and soul of the Ravens, but there were new impact players at just about every position. One young man who stood out almost immediately was Ed Reed.

Ed had a triumphant story of overcoming. Coming from the small Louisiana town of Destrehan, he maximized his moment to become one of the premier safeties to ever play the game. I asked Ed if he could speak to the rookies about being a leader and being professional. He gladly did it and learned the value of leaving a legacy.

I call Ed "Uncle Earl," because he has an old spirit. From his music to his walk, he could easily have lived in the 1970s. He would come by the office and we would just talk about life and whatever was going on. Over the years, Uncle Earl has presented me with three game balls that have meant so much to me.

He often talked about winning a Super Bowl, and when we finally made it to the big game, he presented me with the game ball after the 2013 AFC Championship Game. Ed Reed gave me the greatest gift of all—respect. Now a member of the Houston Texans, I will miss him just coming by the office. As I have learned, assignments are for only a season, but true friendships last a lifetime.

In addition to my work with the Ravens off the field, I got to get back onto the field during practices. I was still in great physical shape and loved the energy and enthusiasm of an early morning practice session with the guys. Rex Ryan, our defensive coordinator, would often ask me to do my best imitation of the opponent the squad was facing the following week.

Sometimes I'd be Jerome Bettis, the running back for the Steelers. Others, I'd be Chad Johnson, the dynamic receiver on the Bengals. If Coach Ryan needed me to pretend I was Peyton Manning, I could do that, too. Or at least, I could try.

"Wherever you need me, Coach." The refrain had worked for me my entire life. If you step up and deliver when called upon—regardless of the task—you'll usually be the one who reaps the benefits in the long run.

After practices, I'd get in the weight room and cut it up with the guys. Some of my best relationships were formed while spotting a player on the bench press or helping him do a new workout routine. Being around the players in that environment on a daily basis kept my competitive spirit alive.

More than anything, though, I enjoyed being someone the guys could rely on. On any day, at any hour, I was available for whatever they needed. Whether it was a talk about a girlfriend—there were several of those—or a hand with finding an internship over the off-season, I wanted the Ravens players to know that I would always be there for them.

Our punter, Sam Koch, likes to remind me of a story from the 2006 season, when Sam was still just a wide-eyed rookie out of the University of Nebraska. He had spent the team's bye week in his hometown with his wife and three kids, and needed a lift from the airport when he got back to Baltimore. He called around, but no one was available to pick him up. When he asked me whether I could grab him, I said, "Of course I'll get you, Sam."

Little did I realize that there'd be a blizzard that night in Baltimore. Sam's flight was scheduled to get in around six p.m., but it was pushed back due to the weather. Chanda and I waited in the BWI Airport parking lot for a few extra hours. It was no problem for us. We enjoyed the peace and quiet, and the snow made for a pleasant backdrop. When midnight rolled around, Sam's flight finally landed.

He called me on his cell phone and started to apologize. "I'll take a cab, O.J. I'm so sorry about that."

"But, Sam, we're in the parking lot waiting for you," I told him.

"You are? You waited for me?"

"Of course I did. That's the Ravens way, my friend," I answered.

On that ride back to Sam's place in Baltimore, he got to know Chanda. We talked about his family, his interests, and his long-term goals and dreams. Sam was a Raven. That meant he was family to Chanda and me. If he ever needed anything—a late-night airport pickup included—he knew he could come to me.

Meanwhile, as I was defining my new role within the organization, Chanda was growing into hers. She served as the Lady Ravens group facilitator, setting up programs and functions for the players' and coaches' wives. We were a team, like we'd always been before, and now we were getting the very most out of our lives by helping those around us.

I was awarded the NFL's Winston/Shell Award in 2005 and 2006, given annually to the player development director who demonstrates commitment in developing innovative ideas to advance the mission of player development. The honor meant a lot, but I knew it was just the start of a great many things to come.

The opportunity—and challenge—of a lifetime lay ahead.

15.

THE NEWS

Consider it pure joy, my brothers and sisters, whenever you face trials of many kinds, because you know
that the testing of your faith produces perseverance.
Let perseverance finish its work so that you may be
mature and complete, not lacking anything.

—James 1:2–4

I picked up the sport of racquetball around the start of the 2005 NFL season. I never played it growing up, but I loved the competitive spirit of the game. After practices, a few of us would head over to the newly built racquetball courts at the Ravens facility and go at it for hours.

After one of these afternoon racquetball sessions during the 2006 season, I felt a strange tingling sensation in my right arm. I assumed it was nothing and put an ice pack on it when I got home. I'd had so many injuries over the course of my career—

whether it was my back, my elbow, or my knees—that a slight tingling didn't strike me as anything out of the ordinary. I knew ex-teammates who were having trouble getting out of bed each morning. Certainly this was nothing to be worried about.

Weeks went by, and the weird feeling in my arm wasn't going away. Instead, it was spreading. After a month or so, I began feeling it in my right shoulder too. I didn't want to alarm anyone at first, and felt some apprehension about it myself, so I didn't do anything about it. Chanda could notice me acting a bit differently and favoring my left hand and arm more than my right around the house, but I did my best to deflect the conversation whenever she'd mention it.

I stopped playing racquetball altogether, and I couldn't perform like I used to in the weight room. The guys on the team even started to notice. Ray Lewis pulled me aside one day after practice and asked whether everything was okay. I assured him it was.

But I really had no idea.

One afternoon, I picked up a football on the practice field and tried throwing it when nobody else was looking. I knew that if I could just throw the football, something I'd done a million times in my life, everything would be okay. But I couldn't. My dexterity was completely off. I could barely even grip the ball.

I knew something wasn't right with my body, but I was hesitant to find out what the problem could be. One night over dinner, I told Chanda about the constant tingling sensation and she urged me to meet with the Ravens team doctor as soon as possible. Of course, she was right. Whereas I'd always been proactive about just about every other aspect of my life—from calling NFL teams on the telephone to pursuing the love of my life—I resisted getting to the bottom of whatever was ailing me. Chanda said she'd come with me on any and all trips to the doctor. She also said that no matter the outcome of the visit, she'd always be by my side. *Always.*

I scheduled a checkup with the team doctors and hoped it was something structural.

We got X-rays done, though, and everything was structurally fine with my body. During my physical, however, the doctors noticed my chest muscles twitching continually, which I would later discover are called fasciculations, a precursor to the muscles starting to break down. They conducted a blood test and the results revealed unusually high levels of glutamate in my bloodstream. Dr. Andrew Tucker, one of the Ravens team physicians, told me this could mean one of two things: I had either contracted Lyme disease or I had something called ALS, amyotrophic lateral sclerosis, more commonly known as Lou Gehrig's disease. Dr. Tucker explained that Lyme could come from a tick bite, but he wasn't as forthcoming about what ALS was or what it could mean.

Whatever was wrong with my body, there was no doubt in my mind that it was merely a temporary condition that I would overcome, just as I had overcome every other adversary that I had faced in my life up until that point. I shared the news with Chanda that afternoon and she felt the natural concern that any spouse would have. I tried to keep her calm, but she was visibly shaken. I told her I'd be fine, but I really had no idea. For the first time since I was a young boy battling my stutter in Houston, I was scared.

The doctors offered me some strengthening exercises and told me to check back in the following weeks.

I did the routines, but nothing seemed to help. My body continued to feel weaker and weaker. This was a much different beast from any of my previous injuries.

Late one sleepless evening, I finally got up out of bed and went on the Internet to look up ALS.

All of my symptoms were there. The tingling. The weakness. The shooting numbness. The muscle cramping. When I noticed the weakness in my right arm, I also experienced a chronic cramping in my right shoulder and my feet. I worked with massage therapists to loosen the muscles, but the cramps would always eventually return.

I enjoyed working out and took great pride in looking like I could still play football, even though those days were long gone. It was about continuing to challenge myself physically. But in less than a year, I went from using 120-pound dumbbells to struggling to press anything at all. The more I read online about ALS, the more I feared I might have the disease.

The biggest shocker from my research was the discovery that ALS was fatal and had a two- to five-year life prognosis from onset.

Hold the phone.

I was just thirty-seven years old.

My body had always been my temple, and I treated it as such. I didn't smoke. I didn't drink. I ate right and was physically active. How could *I* possibly have such a debilitating disease?

I still held out hope that what I had wasn't ALS. I prayed on it. I had seen God deliver me so many times throughout my life. I just knew in the deepest recesses of my heart that He would save me from this as well.

We were referred to a neurologist named Dr. Bruce Rabin in Baltimore, who conducted several nerve conductivity tests. The tests were incredibly uncomfortable and painful. The examination room was just like any ordinary doctor's office, but over in the corner was an odd-looking machine with several dials and wires, with a bottle of blue gel next to it. I recognized the bottle from my training room days as a player. The gel was what we used for ultrasound therapy. However, I didn't recognize the machine, which looked extremely sinister in nature to me.

Dr. Rabin explained the process of the test to me, then began to insert tiny needles into various muscles on my body. Attached to the needles were electrodes that would send electric pulses into my muscles and measure the electrical conductivity of the muscle. The pulses would make my muscles contract involuntarily, and had me sweating like I was going through a workout. I have always had a high pain tolerance, but I wouldn't wish this pain upon my worst enemy. He suspected it might well be ALS, but wouldn't confirm the diagnosis at that point.

Dr. Rabin referred me to Dr. Jeffrey Rothstein, the head of ALS research at the Robert Packard Center, and chair of the neurology department at Johns Hopkins Hospital, for a second opinion. Dr. Rothstein came into the exam room and expressed the usual cordial remarks common to every physician's bedside manner. He reviewed my chart and my nerve conductivity results. He did a few more strength tests on my arms and legs, then recorded the results in my notes.

I really wish God would have given me a vision of the end result of this trial, like He did with my back in Miami, but God was eerily silent that afternoon. This was when I had to rely on the word of God stored inside my spirit instead.

Dr. Rothstein began to share his diagnosis, and my heart sank. As I feared, it was ALS.

The disease impacts roughly six thousand new people worldwide every year. I was now one of those six thousand.

Dr. Rothstein, compassionate and thorough, took us through what was going on. He explained that the human body naturally produces something called glutamate. In ALS, glutamate is not effectively removed from the surface of motor neurons, contributing to further injury and neuronal death.

He made an analogy, describing the motor neurons as telephone wires. In ALS, he said, the signal in the wires doesn't get through to the muscles. As the disease progresses, slowly but surely the muscles deteriorate.

With ALS, he explained, the patient can still think, smell, see, and hear as he or she normally would. The mental capacity is still all there; the physical one, however, is not.

From all of our previous research online, we knew the facts about ALS. I likely had just two to five years left to live. There was a chance I wouldn't see my fortieth birthday. Fifty percent of ALS patients do not live three years beyond the onset of symptoms. Only twenty percent reach five years.

I'd been in peak physical condition just twelve months earlier.

Now I had ALS?

I have always handled bad news fairly well, because God has always shown me the sunshine after the rain. So, as scared as I was, I took the diagnosis with a stiff upper lip. Chanda and I listened to the doctors, and did our best to believe that somehow, someway, we would defy the odds to beat ALS.

I tried to block things out and continue to live my life as I had before hearing the news. Part of it was faith that God would restore me. The other part was just plain old stubbornness and denial.

I put my arm around Chanda and assured her that we'd be okay. Our world had been turned upside down in a matter of weeks, but we were more than capable of facing the future. It wouldn't be easy, but if anyone could take this disease on, it was the two of us.

No one else knew of my diagnosis at the time, but that'd have to change eventually. I thought long and hard about the loved ones around me and struggled with the thoughts of their reactions to the news.

How would Chanda's life change? Would she still be able to pursue her dreams and live her life?

How do you tell your parents that their only son has been diagnosed with ALS?

How do you tell the little sister who's always looked up to you as a pillar of strength that you soon may no longer be able to walk or talk?

How do you explain to your ex-teammates who know you as a weekend warrior that you'll be confined to a motorized chair in the very near future?

These were just a few of the many questions that ran through my head.

I knew I'd take this illness on with a ferocity and vigor it'd never seen before, but how would those who loved me handle the news? The courage to share my illness with others was what I had to dig deep for.

Fortunately, I had Chanda by my side. She was amazing from the very start. She never wavered or looked for a way out. Those first few months were incredibly difficult, but she showed me a strength that I longed to emulate. She had a grasp on what was ahead of us, and she was ready to face that future with me head-on. We'd approach this as we approached everything else in our lives—as a team.

Additionally, I knew I had God to turn to. He'd been watching me my entire life, but I needed Him now more than ever. I knew He was there. He *always* was there.

God told me that nothing in this life is by accident. I'd already seen the impossible accomplished. Having back surgery and being told that there was a chance I was finished, only to be able to heal and come back for the start of the regular season by God's grace—I saw that with my own two eyes. Throughout my life, I continually saw impossibilities overcome. How appropriate that ALS would come on, something that man says is impossible to defeat, and I'd be the one to conquer it. God says all things are possible. I believed it then and still believe it to this day. With God by my side, I believe that regardless of what goes on, I will have a victory. I will overcome.

Chanda and I knew what we were up against. ALS would be the greatest opponent we'd ever faced. We also knew that I was chosen for a reason. "Your whole life has been being told no," Chanda said. "No, you can't play major college football. No, you can't play in the pros. No, you can't make an NFL roster. Every single time, you proved them wrong and you *did* it. Why should this be any different?"

She was right.

Instead of languishing in our misery and continually asking, "Why me?" Chanda and I agreed it was best to ask, "Why *not* me?"

Why *can't* I be the first one to beat this? Just because beating ALS had never been seen before, man seemed to think it was impossible. Well, it was not necessarily impossible; it just hadn't been done *yet*.

The doctors told me the average life span for ALS patients was two to five years after onset, and I could die by the age of forty. Okay. So, what was I going to do about it? Lie down, say, "Woe is me," and cower in a corner for the rest of my life? No. I had to fight. I'd been a fighter my entire life—why stop now? I had to make the most of this opportunity.

And that was truly how I viewed ALS—as an *opportunity*. I'd be the first man to beat ALS, and in the process, I'd raise awareness around the condition. I knew I wasn't alone in this fight. There were thirty thousand others battling the disease, and additional thousands of friends, family, and loved ones impacted by its effects. I had a powerful sphere of influence in my life, and now I had the *opportunity* to make a difference for hundreds of thousands of people.

When I'd get down or upset, Chanda would remind me of a saying: "A man with an outstanding attitude makes the most of it while he gets the worst of it." I'd live by those words. It was my only choice.

Our faith in Jesus gives us a perspective on everything.

It provides me with the understanding that I don't control very much. I do, however, have control over my attitude. I have control over my work ethic. I can control the way I approach life each and every day.

We all deal with a certain form of adversity, and I think it's all in accordance with our faith, as far as what we can handle, and no more will come on us than we can handle. The more I thought about my condition, the more I was encouraged by the opportunities it would provide me.

If I couldn't handle it, God wouldn't allow me to go through it.

16.

IN MY CORNER

It is one of the most beautiful compensations in life that no man can sincerely try to help another without helping himself.

—Ralph Waldo Emerson

WE took time to process everything before we shared the news with anybody.

Once we got our heads around it, we knew it was time to start letting others know. My parents were first.

Chanda and I agreed it was something I had to do in person, no matter how difficult the conversations might be. Telling them was one of the hardest things I've ever done.

Mom and Dad were fighters.

They were just eighteen years old when Mom became pregnant with me. They were married on August 22, 1969. I was born September 29, 1969. Forty-four years after they first met in the spring of 1969, they're still together today.

Dad is the strongest man I know, and the strife he went through as a high school student makes me proud to be his son. He grew up in a tough neighborhood in Houston's First Ward. He came from modest means and learned the importance of punctuality through having no alternatives. If he was the last one to the dinner table at night, he didn't eat.

He was a teenager during the heart of the civil rights era. Due to his high grades and strong character, he was one of the first African-American students to attend the previously all-white Reagan High School. It was a tremendous honor, but also an incredible challenge.

He never wavered, and embraced the opportunity to make history. With that responsibility came wondrous resolve and moments of great hardship. He'd tell me stories of days when he'd be walking the school's hallways and be called racist names by white students who didn't even know him. He was mocked and treated poorly by ignorant kids. In many cases, their parents weren't much better. This was an incredibly trying time in his life, but he looks back on it with pride and a surprising fondness.

"I'd have it no other way, O.J.," he'd tell me. "My personal struggle helped open doors for countless others just like me. I helped change the country."

Many times he'd ignore the spewed hatred and vicious name-calling. Other times he'd fight back. Once, he went to sit down at a lunch table in the school cafeteria and the white children told him he'd have to sit elsewhere. He calmly told them, "No, I am going to sit here," without making much of a spectacle of the situation. They went back and forth with the names and the threats, but he never moved. He didn't leave. One by one, they eventually all got up and sat at another table. He ate his lunch alone that day.

Dad endured this kind of treatment on a regular basis at a young age. He insists that it was good for him, that it made him tougher. It prepared him for life's greater struggles.

There were physical altercations along the way, and sure, he was on the losing side of some of those bouts. But Dad never relented or begged to transfer. He knew of the great responsibility he had as one of the first African-American students in a newly integrated high school. There was no way he was letting that responsibility get the better of him.

Mom was the oldest of four children, and she, too, thrived on responsibility. Her grandparents were the descendants of slaves and played a formidable role in raising her. There was tremendous value placed on hard work and character in her household growing up, and as the eldest sister, she was often in charge of waking her other siblings up in the morning and getting them ready for school. Mom would spend her summers with her cousins in the small town of Alexandria, Louisiana. There she encountered some of the racism and bigotry Dad saw in high school.

In Alexandria, her family members weren't allowed to walk down the same side of the street as the white members of the community. They couldn't eat in the same restaurants or ride on the same public buses. America was a different place back then, and though times were changing, there was still great tension.

Mom's grandparents were responsible for building up her self-esteem at a young age. "They told me that nobody was better than me, and I believed them," she says.

With her mother and father working long hours to provide for the family, she spent a lot of time with her grandma and grandpa. At some point in her teens, she discovered that they both were illiterate. They'd never attended a proper school and hadn't been taught to read or write.

In addition to going to school, caring for her three siblings, and working multiple jobs herself, Mom took on another responsibility as a teenager: She taught her grandma and grandpa how to read and write. It was a painstakingly long process, but Mom wanted them to feel as though they were adjusting as the world changed. As kids, they never dreamed of being able to do such things. She wanted to make that happen for them.

My mother takes great pride in knowing that before they passed, they both learned to read certain words and sign their names. She'd go on to achieve and see a lot in her life, but Mom still views the sight of her grandmother providing her signature on a blank piece of paper as one of her greatest accomplishments.

Mom graduated in the top ten percent of her class. Dad excelled at Reagan High School, too. When she discovered she was pregnant just before their senior prom, they embraced the situation and never saw it as a negative. Rather, they viewed it as a blessing. They also knew what hard work and commitment—to each other—it would take.

After they got married and had me, Mom and Dad got an apartment of their own in the Sunnyside area of Houston, not too far from some other family members.

Dad was hired as a glass cutter and was then later employed by HL&P, the local power company. He started out as a meter reader, but eventually worked his way up to senior-level management in the human resources department. He worked twelve-hour days, earning enough money to make sure food was on the table and his wife and son lived as comfortably as they possibly could. He was a complete man, taking pride in being the first one to work and the last one to punch out.

Most admirable of all, though, was the fact that he went to school at night and received his degree in information technology from the University of Houston while working full-time. He knew a college degree was essential if he was going to make it in corporate America, and he balanced multiple duties—both professionally and personally—to make that happen. The degree didn't come easily, but there was nothing my father couldn't or wouldn't do for his family.

His endless pursuit of the American Dream was matched by my mother's. While raising two kids and holding a full-time job of her own, she also went back to school during her time working at the local phone company. Mom ended up getting her bachelor's degree and worked tirelessly on her master's.

From a young age, they both hustled to make it happen for their family. They made personal sacrifices, but did whatever it took to provide for my sister and me. There was always food on the table and always love in our home.

We were by no means wealthy growing up, but we never felt like we were missing out on anything. We went on family vacations from time to time.

Once, we rented a beach house in the city of Corpus Christi. In Sunnyside, we never saw the ocean or any lakes. This beach house was right on a body of water. Dad wasn't an outdoorsman, and I'd never fished in my life. But the two of us spent hours upon hours that trip, father and son, with fishing rods in hand. He'd tell me stories of his childhood and I'd listen intently. All the while, we just waited for a fish to take the bait.

I don't think we ever caught a single fish that trip, but it didn't matter. We were together, just savoring the time with one another. This was the American Dream, and in my parents' minds, they couldn't imagine anything greater to be achieved.

Through good times and challenging ones, Mom and Dad never gave up on their original agreement to be the best parents they could be. In turn, they provided great lives for my sister and me. Mom and Dad were our biggest fans. No matter their schedules and work commitments, they found a way to be in the stands at every game or track meet they could make, cheering us on. Any honor, any award my sister or I received, Mom and Dad figured out a way to be there, seated in the front row, beaming with pride.

They set the example and served as my role models in life. They inspired me to work hard and to chase my dreams. In turn, I did my very best to accomplish all of the many goals I set for myself to achieve. Playing college football, graduating from Rice, making the NFL, winning a Super Bowl—I'd done everything I'd put my heart, mind, and faith into. I watched Mom and Dad chase the American Dream, but I was truly the embodiment of theirs.

And now I had to board a flight to tell them that their only son—the football star, the scholar, the older brother, the husband, and the man they were always so proud of—had been diagnosed with a life-altering disease for which there was no cure.

Coming to terms with my diagnosis was hard enough, but sharing the news with my parents would be a different sort of obstacle. I knew *I* had the strength to take the disease on, but I needed to find the strength to bring *them* into this new phase of my life. I had to find a way to express to them that I wouldn't be changing. Their son—the hopeless romantic with the Valentine's Day notes in high school, and the man they'd grown to know over the past twenty years—wasn't going anywhere. I'd look different, yes, and my physical capabilities would eventually diminish, but I'd still be their son, O.J. I'd be the same person who was holding that fishing rod with Dad under that simmering sun in Corpus Christi so many years ago. I'd be the same guy who chased down the Giants' kick returner on the first play of Super Bowl XXXV.

I'd be the same person who'd accomplished every goal I ever set for myself. I just needed to communicate all this to my parents. Doing so would take all the courage in the world.

On the phone earlier that week, I told my mother that I was coming back to Houston for a few days and wanted to stop in for dinner with Dad and her at the house. I let her know that there was news I needed to share with them. I booked a round-trip ticket to Houston and I boarded a plane a few days later, as anxious as I'd ever been in my life.

When I got back home to Houston, I went to my childhood home and warmly greeted my folks. Walking through that front door brought back a deluge of childhood memories. Mom has pictures everywhere of my sister and me right through adulthood. I couldn't help but see certain pictures and notice how I had changed over the years. Unfortunately, there was another change coming.

We went into the kitchen and sat at the same table where I ate just about every meal as a kid. As Mom, Dad, and I engaged in small talk, I was distracted by the thought of the conversation we'd soon be having. I'd played out the discussion in my head a hundred times over the past forty-eight hours, but I still didn't know how it would go. I didn't even know where to start.

How do you tell your parents that their child could be dead within a matter of years? In the natural order of life, children are supposed to outlive their parents, not the other way around.

Eventually, I shared with them the news of my diagnosis.

My folks took it very hard, but I tried to assure them that Chanda and I would be okay and fully expected to beat the disease. Dad tried to comfort Mom as she wept bitterly, but there was no comfort to be had. I had always been a mama's boy, but I emphasized to my father that I needed *him* now more than ever. He always seemed to have a calm demeanor no matter what was going on, and I wanted to draw from that strength in my fight against ALS. Just like Chanda and I needed time to process everything, so did they.

Dad asked me to leave the room for a moment while they took time to understand it all. I felt awful for making Mom cry.

They'd always been there for me, providing solutions to

problems and alternative outlooks on things whenever I had doubts or was feeling down. In this instance, they had no magical wand to wave to make everything better. But they did what I hoped they would—they lent their unwavering support and believed in me. I told them I was going to beat ALS, and they never questioned my will. My father's first words to me after I told him the news were, "We'll beat this thing."

We. I loved that.

"O.J.," he said with his hand now on my shoulder, "you've overcome every obstacle you've ever faced in your life. You've never ceased to amaze the two of us. If you say you're going to beat ALS, then yes, you're going to beat ALS. We'll be with you every step of the way. Every single step."

My mother dried her eyes and hugged me tightly. "We love you," she said. "We're in this together. Whatever you need from us, wherever you need us—we're here for you, son."

The three of us said a prayer and agreed that God would see us through.

The conversation, though incredibly difficult, went about as well as I could have possibly imagined. The end result—my parents in my corner, by my side for the fight of my life—was everything I could have asked for.

My little sister was next.

17.

BIG BRO

Do not be anxious about anything, but in every situation, by prayer and petition, with thanksgiving, present your requests to God. And the peace of God, which transcends all understanding, will guard your hearts and your minds in Christ Jesus.

—Philippians 4:6–7

WHEN I was four years old and my mother was eight and a half months pregnant, I announced at a family reunion that if the baby was a boy, I wanted it sent back.

"Return it," I instructed.

I simply had no interest in competing with *another* man in the house.

Fortunately, my parents didn't have to address my demand. Myla Brigance was born in December of 1973, and she's the greatest Christmas gift I've ever received. I loved my little sister right from the start.

Though we fought like cats and dogs throughout our entire childhood, we were also always the best of friends. Myla mimicked and copied everything I did. It was fun having a partner in crime, even if she was four years my junior, and I tolerated her often wearing the same clothes, talking the same way, and making the same funny faces as me. The two of us would stand on the corner of our block for hours on end, trying to lure crawfish out of ditches with bologna on sticks. It was mindless entertainment, but Myla and I could do it forever. As long as we were out there together, we were having fun.

I knew when I was ten years old that Myla would always have my back. I was rude to my mother at the dinner table one night and was grounded for a week. I wasn't too happy with the punishment and came up with an alternative course of action: I decided I'd run away.

I had no idea where I was going to go, but I was ready to explore. I packed a bag with clean underwear, a few pairs of pants, and some T-shirts. I *may* have packed a toothbrush, too. I may not have. Either way, I was leaving. As I was getting ready for my great escape, my six-year-old sister saw me putting my belongings in my overnight bag.

"Where are you going?" she asked curiously.

"I don't know," I told her.

"Can I come, too?"

I thought about it for a few moments. What good would the adventure be if I didn't have Myla to share it with?

"Sure!"

She quickly ran to the garage, got a big paper grocery bag of her own, and started packing her clothes, too. I got our bikes—mine a Huffy, hers a pink one with training wheels—and put them out in the front yard. In the kitchen, I made two peanut butter–and-jelly sandwiches for the road. Like cat burglars in the night, we were ready to sneak away. Where were we going? We really had no idea.

At the last second, before the big escape, I got scared. It wasn't particularly safe after hours where we lived, and we had no business being outside the house. I told Myla to go say good-bye to Mom and Dad, who were getting ready for bed. When a six-year-old girl says, "Mommy, Daddy—we're running away," your cover is pretty much blown. Mom came out into the kitchen, saw me with my fully packed bag and lunchbox full of PB&J sandwiches, and couldn't help but laugh.

"Go to bed, O.J.," she said with a smile.

Myla, my little coconspirator, was disappointed. She was ready for an adventure. To this day, she insists that she would have left with me that night. Anywhere. Anytime. Anything to be with her big brother. It's always been that way. I love her for that.

As we got older, I grew into a protective older brother. No boy was ever good enough for my little sister. She'd date guys in high school and I'd scoff at their haircuts, mock the way they spoke, or criticize the dates they took her on. I was in college, but I always kept tabs on Myla and the boys courting her. My father wasn't a man to be messed with, but those high school boys feared me a lot more than they did my dad.

Though she was one of the more popular girls in her grade, she asked *me* to be her date or chaperone to most of her high school functions. I always obliged.

And I was always a goofball. To her junior prom, I wore a top hat, a suede jacket, and flip-flops. I was her date to her debutante ball, too. She was crowned the debutante and had to do the customary waltz after having the crown placed upon her head. There we were, brother and sister, in a beautiful hotel ballroom, *waltzing* to an Anne Murray song.

I'd always ask Myla why she didn't just go with boys her age. Her answer was always the same: "I figured I'd have more fun with you."

And fun we had.

I'd eventually let Myla live her own life, though. There comes a time when you—even as the big brother—have to let go.

When she was in college at Texas Christian University, she was a star on the track-and-field squad. She fell hard for a boy on the football team, and I remember having my reservations. I *was* a football player. I'd been in those locker rooms my entire life. I didn't like the thought of Myla being the subject of any locker room chatter, but I stayed quiet. A few months after they started dating, they began having issues. I told her to break up with the guy.

"Don't ever date football players. They're bad news," I insisted.

"But *you're* a football player," she answered back, on the defensive.

"But I'm different!"

Myla grew up to be a beautiful and accomplished woman. She's a business owner now, the mother of three wonderful children, and is married to a great man and father.

Though surrounded by it her entire life, Myla didn't understand the rules to football and never bothered to learn them. The fact that she traveled the world to see me compete at every level, despite having no particular interest in the game, says a lot about her. Myla flew to Seattle and drove to Vancouver to see me play in the Canadian Football League. She made the trip to Miami when I first suited up for the Dolphins. When I was playing for the Ravens in Super Bowl XXXV down in Tampa Bay, Myla bought a plane ticket to be in town for the weekend.

If I ever came across as overly protective of her, it was merely a by-product of how important she is to me. She would groan at having her big brother meddling in her personal life, and then thank me for being a shoulder to cry on.

Now I needed *her* to be strong.

Shortly after speaking with my parents, I told Myla about my diagnosis. She took the news incredibly hard. I'd always been her "big bro," an invincible force and her great protector. Now I was telling her the details of my condition, and she was having trouble envisioning me in my future state.

She told me she loved me, but I could tell there was a great amount of fear and sadness in her eyes. She said she'd noticed me struggling to lift her daughter the last time I was with her in Texas, but assumed it was the result of an old football injury. She didn't want to think of any possible alternatives. "Myla, I'm going to be okay," I told her. "I promise."

I'd never broken a promise to my little sister in my life, and I didn't plan on doing it now.

She struggled with the news and began to well up. It took all the strength I had inside of me to not break down with her. "I'm not going anywhere, Myla," I reiterated. "I'm going to beat this. Trust me. I will."

She'd never seen me weak or vulnerable. To my younger sister, I was always the model of strength. This was going to be a very difficult transition for her to endure, but it was one that I simply couldn't control. I asked her to pray with me and to be by my side. She said she'd always be there for me, like she'd been throughout our lives.

That's all I wanted.

18.

TEAMMATES FOR LIFE

What counts in life is not the mere fact that we have lived. It is what difference we have made to the lives of others that will determine the significance of the life we lead.

—Nelson Mandela

BEYOND Mom, Dad, Myla, and Chanda, I kept the news of my illness to myself at first. I knew I had to tell my employers at some point, but struggled to find the right moment. I became visibly thinner and weaker as the disease progressed, and many of the players and coaches were beginning to notice. The time to let the organization know of my diagnosis had come.

I headed to Ravens training camp in Westminster, Maryland, in August of 2007 with great apprehension. A series of questions ran through my head. Would the Ravens still want me around? How would the guys react to the news? Would I serve as a distraction?

On the first day of camp, I knocked on the door of Coach Billick's temporary office at McDaniel College. He was just getting settled for another NFL campaign, and I knew how focused he was during this time of year. The last thing I wanted to do was bother him.

"Coach Billick, do you have a second?" I asked him.

He didn't lift his head from his paperwork, and responded, "What's up, Juice?"

"Well," I began, my stomach in knots, "I wanted to tell you about an amazing opportunity I've been blessed with. An opportunity that is going to change my life forever."

Coach Billick put down his pen and slowly lifted his head. I could tell he was a bit taken aback. Here it was, the start of the NFL's busiest time of the year, and I was coming to him about some sort of new opportunity.

"Well, what's the new job, Juice? Which team's front office are you leaving us for?"

I smiled. "No, Coach. No new team. No new job. I've been blessed with an opportunity far greater than that."

I took a deep breath.

"Coach, I have ALS," I said. "God has challenged me with another test, and I'm going to take the disease on. I have been given the opportunity to be the first person to conquer ALS. And I will."

Coach Billick got up from behind his desk and approached me. He wrapped both of his arms around me and held me close to him. He, too, had noticed my health deteriorating over the past year. "I love you, Juice," he told me. "The Ravens will support you in your battle and will do whatever you need."

His words were not empty. When the news spread to the front office and the team's owners, the outpouring of love and support was unfathomable. Ozzie Newsome told me I'd have a job with the team for as long as I wanted, and offered to hire me a full-time assistant to help with the director of player programs role. Harry Swayne, an ex-teammate of mine on the 2000 Ravens, was hired to work alongside me. Dick Cass, the president of the organization since 2004, told me, "We are honored to stand beside you, O.J. Your courage and fire are remarkable. You're a Raven for life."

Owner Steve Bisciotti went out of his way to do everything in his power to help Chanda and me in our fight against ALS. He insisted, "What's mine is yours," without ever providing me an opportunity to decline his graciousness. He helped ensure we'd have the top medical care in the world and access to everything we could have ever asked for. Art Modell, the team's longtime owner, asked Chanda and me what he and his wife could do to help, too. "Anything," he said, "Anything at all. Just say the word." Whether it was Coach Billick, Ozzie, Dick, Steve Bisciotti, or Art Modell—they all were willing to drop everything at any given moment to support Chanda and me.

They all echoed the same sentiments I'd shared with Sam Koch when I'd picked him up from the airport a few months earlier. They exemplified the Ravens way.

It was time to share the news with the guys. I decided to wait until we got back from training camp, and addressed the entire team in front of the auditorium at the facility in Owings Mills, Maryland.

"Men, a lot of you have probably noticed that I've lost some weight and haven't looked the same over the past few months," I said. "There's a reason for that. I've been diagnosed with ALS, also known as Lou Gehrig's disease."

I explained that I would eventually lose all mobility, and possibly my life. I could see that they were visibly concerned and shaken. I assured them all that I would fight this demon with every ounce of my being and that I would win the fight. I encouraged them to lift up their heads and to stand with me.

"I can tell by looking at some of your eyes that when you saw me today or yesterday, you looked at me differently, because I look different than you saw a month ago or two months ago. Don't be afraid. Don't be afraid to be close to me. Don't be afraid to witness what you're witnessing."

I concluded, "I want you all to know right now that I *will* beat this disease. I have no doubts about that. It might be a struggle, but I will be victorious. I believe I'll be the one to beat ALS. If there is one, I'll be the one. I don't want you to pity or feel any bit of sorrow about this news. If anything, I want to thank all of you for your drive and your pride. Watching you Mighty Men go to battle inspires *me* every day."

Ray and Ed both made their way to the front of the auditorium. Ray kissed me on my head and hugged me as tightly as he ever had before. Ed patted me on my back and nodded his head in agreement. I demanded that neither one of them ever treat me any differently than they did before I was diagnosed. I looked in Ray's eyes and told him I was going to beat this thing. He never had any doubt that I would. "We've had a special relationship since day one, Juice. You know that," he said. "I looked to you for support in my time of need and you were there. You've always inspired me. I won't treat you any differently than I did the first day we met. I promise."

Clutching him, I felt his love. "And I know you'll beat this," he said. "Of course you'll beat this. We're going to beat this *together*, Juice."

Ed echoed similar sentiments and joined the hug.

They are both great, great men. They are my brothers.

My one request to every person in the Ravens organization was to not treat me any differently than they had before. The guys would always joke with me and give me shout-outs when they walked by my office door. I didn't want that to change. I knew those shout-outs would serve as both therapy and my greatest weapon against ALS.

I asked of them only one thing: normalcy. If the guys could give me that, I'd be okay.

Rex Ryan came by my office a few minutes after I shared the news with the team, and encouraged me by saying, "If anyone can beat this, O.J., it's you." I'd known Rex for nearly a decade. I played for him and now worked alongside him every day. His words meant a lot.

The rest of the guys exhibited their love for me through their actions. One morning when I got to the facility, all of the parking spaces near the entrance of the building were taken. I parked in the back of the lot and began my walk into work. Midway through, my shoulder grew weak and I was forced to put my bag down and collect myself.

Derrick Mason, our number one wide receiver at the time, was leaving the facility to go home and saw me struggling on his way out. Derrick didn't say a single word. He didn't ask any questions or embarrass me by calling attention to my circumstances. Instead, he parked his car, got out, and walked me all the way inside the building and into my office. He placed my bag on the floor and asked whether I needed anything else. I thanked Derrick for the assistance, but he wouldn't have it. "Have a great day, O.J.," he said with a smile. He left the room and never mentioned it to anyone.

The most impressive thing to me was that the guys never gave pity, which would have been degrading. Instead, they stood in the gap, ready to help me fight.

After telling my immediate family and my Ravens family of my diagnosis, it was time to share the news with the rest of my inner circle. I let Todd, Karl, and ex-teammates like Larry Izzo, Zach Thomas, Qadry Ismail, and Danny Barrett know about my illness in the following months. None of them batted an eye. The more people I told, the more encouraged I was about the prospects of my ALS journey. My circle of influence rallied around me and lifted me to new heights. Their positivity, their love, and their collective good spirits encouraged me to believe I could continue to live my life and do whatever I wanted—despite what the medical data said.

They were all in my corner. Every last one of them said they'd battle ALS *with* me, and lend their support in any way possible. They've all been there by my side every single step of the way.

What a great relief it was to know I wasn't alone in my fight. Chanda was the driving force, and I had an incredible group of friends and family willing to attack this disease with the same ferocity I was. The Ravens organization, in particular, lent their support and encouragement in a way I couldn't possibly have imagined. God was watching over all of us.

I was now energized by the bout ahead. How could I not be? I had an amazing group of fighters in my corner.

19.

GETTING THROUGH

One word frees us of all the weight and pain of life:
That word is love.

—Sophocles

I eventually lost the ability to hold a pen.

My dexterity became clumsier, too, making it a monumental task to make knots for my ties or put on my pants in the morning. One day after work, I was trying to unbutton my shirt with my left arm. Chanda wasn't home at the time, so I lay on the bed to get a better angle on the buttons. I wrestled with them for more than an hour and a half. It was as exasperating a moment in my life as I can remember. I was driven to tears because I couldn't complete this simple task that I'd done a million times before. Agitated and worn out after struggling with my shirt for so long, I ultimately gave up and took a nap, fully clothed.

When Chanda returned home that night, she assisted me in

getting undressed. I thanked her, but remained in a funk for the remainder of the evening.

The initial stages of my bout with ALS were the toughest for me, because I still had my independence, but daily tasks like eating, brushing my teeth, and dialing the phone were becoming increasingly more difficult. I had made a living relying on my body, and now I felt as though it was betraying me.

The inability to do the most routine things was the hardest part of the illness to come to terms with. You take for granted being able to comb your hair and tie your own shoes. I could no longer do either.

I did my best to block out all of the negativity and self-pity, but every day became more and more arduous. One evening I hit a low point. I was sitting at the kitchen table with Chanda when the weight of the diagnosis came crashing down on me. I don't recall what, if anything, triggered it, but suddenly the grim reality of the situation took hold of both of us.

"Do you mean I could be dead by the age of forty and there is really nothing I can do about it?" I asked aloud. "Nothing? There's no cure, Chanda? Nothing?!"

I broke down and started to cry. Chanda joined me. We cried and cried, letting all of our emotions out right there at our kitchen table. I'm not sure Chanda had ever seen me cry before, but there was no embarrassment. No machismo to protect. The tears poured out of both of us simultaneously as we held each other tight. The great unknown, the utter lack of control over the future, and the fragility of life hit us all at once.

After a few minutes, we both dried our tears. Our spirits were reminded of God's words: "Never will I leave you or forsake you."

It was time to find the purpose for the pain.

20.

MAKING ADJUSTMENTS

I can accept failure; everyone fails at something. But I can't accept not trying.

—Michael Jordan

AS ALS continued to ravage my body, it became increasingly difficult to do more and more things. I was told that this would happen, but I faced every new physical challenge with an obstinate heart. I hoped the disease progression would slow down or stop altogether, so I continued to push myself. But several incidents during my first year with ALS forced me to make some adjustments. If I didn't change the way I was approaching the disease, I was going to end up really hurting myself.

I enjoyed the opportunity to travel with the team on the road throughout the 2007 season. Usually we would depart Baltimore the day before a Sunday game and board the plane a couple of hours after the game was over to return home. The schedule is very tight and moves at a fast pace. One week, we were deplaning and it was raining cats and dogs. By the time I finally got my bags together, everybody else had already unloaded the aircraft and boarded the buses. I had only one good arm to hold my umbrella and my bag, and the wind was blowing hard. It was such a struggle to navigate the stairs and carry everything in a timely fashion. The entire team was waiting on me, but I was too proud to ask for help. It took me fifteen minutes to get from the plane to the bus.

That evening marked the first time that I felt like deadweight and a hindrance to the rest of the guys. I was interrupting the routine, and in sports, that could be the difference between winning and losing. I finally made it onto the bus, but realized my days of traveling with the team would soon be over.

Driving was also becoming increasingly more difficult. When my right arm lost its strength and dexterity, I began driving solely with my left hand. It became a real process to start the car, and making turns was problematic. This period of my life was incredibly difficult for me, because I absolutely loved driving. I grew up waiting for the opportunity to get my driver's license and, ultimately, my independence. Some of my favorite times were spent in my old red Duster or the Ford Explorer. I loved being behind the wheel, music blasting, with nothing but the open road in front of me.

Those days would soon come to an end, too.

One afternoon I was driving through a roundabout traffic circle and couldn't turn the wheel fast enough, almost causing a major accident. The incident scared me, but not to the point that I would give up driving just yet. I continued on, denying the obvious fact that I'd have to put down the keys at some point.

A few weeks later, Darren Sanders, the Ravens director of security, and Harry Swayne, the assistant director of player development, came into my office to speak to me. I could tell something was up, but didn't know what was coming. Harry knelt next to me and expressed their shared concern about me driving myself to and from work every day. I soon discovered what was going on: This was an intervention. I politely listened, but inside I was very upset with both of them. How could they ask me to give up driving? Didn't they realize that this was more than just getting to and from a destination? Didn't they realize that it symbolized independence?

Though deep down I knew I was endangering myself and the lives of countless others every time I got behind the wheel, I saw giving up the keys as a sign of defeat. With every freedom I lost, I viewed it as ALS getting the best of me. I viewed it as ALS winning the fight.

Their sit-down initially angered me, but I really appreciated the love Harry and Darren showed in broaching the subject. They loved me. They were only coming from a place of concern and deep emotion. The Ravens graciously offered to hire me a driver to take me wherever I needed to go, and I accepted.

The team has been with us every step of the way to make this situation easier. We so love and appreciate them for that. Because Steve Bisciotti and the Ravens were such a blessing to us, we wanted to be a blessing to others. That was when the light really turned on for Chanda and me. It was when we decided to use my platform to bring greater awareness to ALS.

21.

NEW FRIENDS

Even if I knew that tomorrow the world would go to
pieces, I would still plant my apple tree.

—Martin Luther

FOLLOWING the 2007 season, the Ravens replaced Brian Billick with John Harbaugh as the team's new head coach. I was familiar with John's name because he was the longtime special teams assistant for the Philadelphia Eagles under Andy Reid. Special teams guys know other special teams guys. In a way, we're all members of a fraternity within the fraternity of NFL players.

The first day I met him, John grabbed my hand and shook his head. "Man, O. J. Brigance," he said. "It's an honor to meet you. We used to watch tapes of you and Larry Izzo when you two played in Miami. You guys were like cheetahs in the wild out there."

I knew right from the start that I'd like this guy. A little flattery goes a long way. It just so happens that Harbs and I had a lot more in common than a mutual admiration for each other's careers. He was a devout Christian family man who lived his life the right way. His love for his wife, Ingrid, and his daughter, Alison, knew no bounds. He also placed great value on quality of character and hard work. His Ravens team would emulate their head coach. They'd be hardworking, smart, and prepared to take on adversity.

A new head coach can mean a lot of things in the NFL. One of them is turnover. John had every opportunity to replace the "old regime" with his own guys. But from the very start, he told me that my job was safe as long as he was in the building. He asked me to be as present as I possibly could, and told me that he wanted his players to follow my lead.

From the first day Ozzie introduced us, I saw John's energetic passion for the people and the game he's loved since he was a boy. When I met his dad, Jack Harbaugh, I saw where his sense of integrity came from. The influence of Mr. Harbaugh was evident, but there was something else—a peaceful calmness, with an ear to hear what God was saying in the moment. John and I formed a special relationship based on our mutual love for Jesus Christ. He took every opportunity to include me as part of the team as completing my day-to-day duties became increasingly more difficult. We would spend time talking about how we could make the guys and the team stronger through building stronger relationships.

I'd drop John notes when I woke up, often encouraging him to keep fighting the good fight or to share a passage from the Bible that I found particularly relevant. In return, he'd offer his words of inspiration or make a joke to lighten my day. I'd grow to rely on John's e-mails as a source of great happiness. To this day, a smile comes across my face when I see one of his morning messages awaiting me in my in-box.

Though I could no longer participate in practices like I used to, I made a point to still be on the sideline for each and every one of them. If it was raining or snowing, it didn't matter—I was going to be there. That didn't change when I lost the ability to walk. I'm still out there every day, observing things from my spot next to Ozzie Newsome, watching practice and taking mental notes.

Harbs wanted a team of fighters. He liked guys who had chips on their shoulders and something to prove. He sought out players who thrived when they were doubted. His first two draft picks were the perfect fit for the team he was building in Baltimore.

Joe Flacco was a six-foot-six-inch quarterback who simply never took no for an answer. When he was told he'd be the backup and have to wait at least a year to get his opportunity to start at the University of Pittsburgh, he transferred to Delaware, a Division I-AA school where he knew he'd get the chance to shine right away. At Delaware he flourished, but was knocked by NFL draft "experts" for putting up big numbers against what was considered lesser competition. When the Ravens selected him in the first round of the 2008 NFL draft, there were questions as to whether he'd be ready to make the jump from a lesser-known college football program to the NFL. It was a familiar story that I knew all too well.

In the second round of the '08 draft, the Ravens selected Ray Rice out of Rutgers. Ray was a record-breaking running back for the Scarlet Knights in college, but was passed over by thirty-two NFL teams (including the Ravens) in the first round of the NFL draft because of his size. He was just five-foot-eight, and there were doubts he'd ever make it in the pros. I'd heard that one before, too.

I met both Ray and Joe the day after they were drafted. Joe arrived at the Ravens facility in a button-down shirt and slacks, with his mother, father, and girlfriend (now his wife), Dana, by his side. When he was first introduced to me, he grabbed for my hand and attempted to give me a firm handshake. My arm, at the time, however, had lost most of its strength. Joe hesitated for a moment, let go of my hand, and took a nervous step backward.

"Just grab it," I instructed.

"Yeah?" Joe asked, trying not to hurt or injure me.

"Yes. Just grab it. I'll be okay. I promise."

Joe took hold of my hand and gave me a firm handshake. "All right, then," he said with a grin.

I let Joe know my role with the team and showed him and his family around the facility. I also told him, "You're going to have a lot on your plate this year. I'm not going to get in your way. Just know that I will always be here for you."

Ray, Joe, and I hit it off when I took their 2008 rookie class to the NFL's Rookie Symposium in San Diego that summer. It was a great trip, and a time when I got to know both of them very well. In turn, they got to know me and what I was all about. I'll always remember Joe and Ray as wide-eyed rookies, but they've each grown so much in the five years I've known them.

Joe won the starting quarterback job in training camp that summer and hasn't missed a single start in his five-year NFL career. Ray played running back, sharing carries with veteran Willis McGahee in the backfield. An elder Ray on the squad took an immediate liking to the new Ray and placed him under his wing. Ray Lewis and Ray Rice were an inseparable duo, going as "Ray and Li'l Ray" around the facility. Midway through the season, someone dubbed them Mufasa and Simba, based on the father and son characters in the Disney movie *The Lion King*. Ray Lewis served as a mentor for Li'l Ray, getting him involved in the team's Bible-study sessions and community activities. He also showed him how hard you have to work if you want to make it in this league. Watching their relationship flourish over the course of five seasons has been one of the most rewarding parts of my job with the team. Li'l Ray would eventually grow to be quite the team leader himself.

Prior to the start of the 2008 regular season, Coach Harbaugh asked me whether I'd be willing to address the team. I asked him for a few days to prepare something and wrote a speech. Before practice one afternoon that summer, the team gathered in front of me. I collected myself and read the following:

> My Mighty Men,
>
> It was about a year ago that I stood before you and let you all know that I had ALS. Circumstances don't determine outcomes, gentlemen. As I saw on many of your faces when you saw me coming back, things have changed a little bit, huh?
>
> First of all, I want to apologize to you, because you are going to have to go through something that no other team in the NFL will have to endure. You will have to see a man walk out before you into possible death. That can be tough and scary for some people. Now, I say "possible" because I still believe that I will be healed. Regardless of what it looks like, believe me, my spirit is still strong. Understand that every bit of what we're going to give you . . . time is precious.
>
> Do not make the mistake of thinking that this is just another training camp. No matter how long you've been in this league, make no mistake in understanding that you are blessed to be in this room.

Many people who look at me will turn their head because they just can't bear to look. But I want to encourage you, men, to look at me and understand that you have a tremendous opportunity. Opportunity to live, to play a game that no one else has the opportunity to play. For those of you who are privileged to make this team, you will see something walk out before you that no other team will have an opportunity to experience. And from that, you will get an opportunity to see what true courage is.

I want you to understand something. Many have said, "I don't know if I could do that, if I could go through that, if I could handle that." You could. I'm not strong. I'm as weak as every one of you. But because of my faith, I know that I'm going to be okay, regardless.

I'm going to work it out day by day. There may be some hot days. Someone may blow out their knee. They are out. Adversity. Men, each and every one of you deal with something in your life that challenges you, and it is going to continue to be that way, because we live in a world where not everything goes perfectly.

I want to encourage you, every time you look at me, every time you see Harry, understand that we are here for you. Do not give in to your circumstances. Do not give in to the heat, do not give in to weariness, do not give in to soreness, and, if you do that, you will have something special before it is all said and done.

I say this, fellas, not for an ovation, not for any type of admiration, but because I am a man just like you are. There are things that you are probably dealing with that I wouldn't even know how to help you with. But we also want you to know that because of our experiences, we can walk that walk with you. We are going to give you everything that we've got. Men, it is going to be a great year. Don't accept anything less.

22.

THE WALK OF A LIFETIME

You may encounter many defeats, but you must not be
defeated. In fact, it may be necessary to encounter the
defeats, so you can know who you are, what you can
rise from, how you can still come out of it.

—Maya Angelou

ONE of my proudest moments as an older brother came on July
21, 2008. My sister, Myla, was marrying Terry Gabriel, the love
of her life. They rented a gorgeous room in a restaurant called
Maggiano's in Houston and had all of their closest friends and
family members by their sides.

The flowers, the music, and the weather were all perfect. It
was truly a celebration of their love.

Right before the ceremony began, Myla pulled me aside and
did me the ultimate honor.

She asked me to take her down the aisle and present her to our father.

I was now roughly a year and a half into my battle with ALS and had been having a particularly difficult time of late. There are good days and there are bad days when confronting this condition. I recall the few months leading up to Myla's wedding as incredibly tough ones, both emotionally and physically. I had already lost most of the use of my arms, and now my legs were growing weaker, too. Having dropped so much weight in the previous few months, I knew it'd be startling for some of our family members attending the wedding to see me in my condition. In the days leading up to the event, I didn't sleep very much. I just wanted to be at my very best on Myla's special day.

Her request to walk her down the aisle gave me a purpose, and instead of being anxious about my ability to perform, I was confident. There was simply no way I wasn't going to make that walk with my sister on my arm. The thought of her relying on me—despite my current condition—comforted me in a way she'd never know. At that moment, Myla wasn't viewing me as stricken with an illness. She was viewing me as her big brother, the rock who always protected and looked out for her best interests.

As the music played, she emerged and glided into the room. She looked beautiful in her white dress. I looked her in the eyes and we both smiled. I'd be lying if I didn't say I was welling up with tears.

Step. Breathe.

Step. Breathe.

Step. Breathe.

She held on to my arm and I held on to her. At that moment, we were same O.J. and Myla who used to hunt for crawfish in ditches down in Sunnyside. Any fears or trepidation I had leading up to the weekend were now gone.

I was walking just fine. God was lifting us both on the most memorable of days. When I got Myla to my father, the three of us quickly embraced and I returned to my seat.

I prepared a few words for later on in the evening, but I wasn't sure I'd have the courage to deliver them when the moment came to do so. In addition to my arms and legs, my voice was beginning to weaken now, too. I'd been told it was going to happen, but the realization was incredibly hard.

When I was asked to address the newly married couple, I found an inner strength that gave me the ability to project for the entire room to hear.

I told Myla how happy I was for her and Terry. I told her how proud of her I was. I made a few jokes. I said some words from the heart. I told her that no matter what she did or where she went, I'd always be by her side.

"I love you, sis," I finished.

It was one of the very last times my family heard me speak before I fully lost the ability to use my voice.

I'm forever grateful I had the opportunity to say all the things that I'd wanted to tell Myla that evening.

That was one of my favorite nights of my life.

23.

CLIMBING THE MOUNTAIN

Don't worry about failures; worry about the chances
you miss when you don't even try.

—Jack Canfield

MY health steadily worsened over the course of that 2008 season. My legs and my balance weakened and caused a few bad falls, the worst of which landed me in the emergency room to get nine stitches above my eye. A hard head makes a soft behind, my folks used to say. Well, I finally got it through my thick skull that I should use my wheelchair more, for my safety.

I dreaded the wheelchair at first.

I would stare at it with contempt, because it symbolized restriction. I would try to stand and walk as much as I could, until I would get too exhausted to stay on my feet any longer. This was a tough transition period, because I saw it as further evidence that my body was deteriorating instead of healing.

I'd lost much of the use of my arms and legs by midseason and was forced to use the motorized wheelchair to get around the facility on a regular basis.

It was a difficult time, but the team inspired me to battle every day. Watching them work together as one toward a unified goal gave me hope and served as a reason to get out of bed in the morning. There was a job to do and they were doing it. I merely followed their lead.

I turned to God, too. When times got particularly difficult, I didn't ask, "Why?" or grow overly frustrated. I relied on God to show me the way. There was a reason for all of this, a greater purpose. I knew it. I just needed to be as strong as I possibly could be and do what Danny Barrett always advised: I needed to press on.

We went 11–5 during the regular season, securing a postseason berth in John's, Joe's, and Ray's first years with the team. In the wild-card round of the play-offs, we traveled to Miami and beat the Dolphins, my former team, behind four interceptions from our defense. Ed Reed took one back sixty-one yards for a touchdown.

The following week, we made the trip to Tennessee, where we faced the top seeded Titans in their building. Though we were big underdogs, we never doubted that we could take Tennessee down if we played our game. I traveled to Tennessee and watched the battle from my motorized chair in the press box. It was an old-school slugfest, filled with hard hitting and very little offense. In other words, it was just the type of game I always loved. When it was all said and done, the Mighty Men pulled off another upset.

After the win, I made a point to be standing on my feet when the guys walked into the locker room, victorious. I hadn't been walking very much around the facility of late, but I wanted to show the team my strength. I wanted to show them that I could still get up and rise to the occasion—just like them.

Losing the ability to walk was one of the hardest things I'd ever faced in my life. For years as a football player, I relied on three things: my heart, my mind, and my legs. Though I was never the biggest guy in the locker room or the most feared tackler on the field, my speed always made me a dynamic football player. Whether it was running that 4.57 forty-yard dash for Jimmy Johnson in 1996 or chasing down countless kick returners as a Ravens special teams ace, I knew I always could count on my legs.

Now I could no longer run.

I could barely walk.

I couldn't do all the things that I once had been able to do, but I knew I *could* do one thing.

I could still stand.

And that evening in that locker room in Nashville, I made a point to be on my two feet when those Mighty Men walked through the doors. Any physical pain would have to be blocked out. If the Ravens could rally around one another and knock off the number one seeded Titans, I could certainly overcome my temporary discomfort and stand among them. What they had just accomplished on the football field motivated me to silence the doubts in my head and to stand tall.

Joe Flacco, now just one win away from a Super Bowl in his rookie year, grabbed my hand firmly when he entered the locker room and said, "Juice! Great to see you up out of the chair!"

Joe had all the confidence in the world. He wasn't scared of the unknown, and he certainly was no longer scared of shaking my hand as hard as he could. I was extremely proud of the way he played that afternoon.

Terrell Suggs, our dynamic linebacker, couldn't finish the

game due to an injury he suffered in the second half. Ozzie asked him whether he thought he'd be able to go the following week. Terrell pointed over in my direction. "I see O.J. standing," he said. "I'll be out there next week. I'll be fine."

Coach Harbaugh gathered the team in the locker room and presented the game ball to Ed Reed, who'd had another fabulous effort. Ed, in turn, pointed my way.

"Game ball, baby," Ed said as he handed the ball over to me. "The last one they threw, man. To O.J., baby."

Ed put the ball in my hands and patted me on the head. "We love you, O.J.," he said.

I looked around the room and saw the Mighty Men beaming back at me. Harbs was nodding his head, and guys like Brendon Ayanbadejo and Samari Rolle were chanting, "Juiiiiiiiiice!"

I was on my feet, but I might as well have been floating on air. The room was electric. My speech was very slurred at the time, but I found the inner strength to deliver a message loud and clear. The love of the Mighty Men empowered me.

"All things are possible," I began. "We've been saying it. All things are possible. If you don't give in to your circumstances, you won't believe where you'll find yourself. You didn't give in and you never stopped swinging. That's all right."

"Yeah," shouted one of the guys.

"It ain't over," I continued. "It ain't over. God has a higher purpose and a higher plan. Don't be satisfied, and don't celebrate too much. We've got some more work to do."

I looked at Coach Harbaugh and our owner, Steve Bisciotti, as they both nodded their heads and pumped their fists.

But I wasn't finished. My voice got even stronger, and any discomfort I felt from standing was numbed by the beautiful positive energy in the room.

"One vision. One focus. For a higher purpose, men. Don't forget. Don't forget it. I didn't want to be in that chair when you all walked in here. I don't want to be in that chair. I will walk again, and we *will* be champions."

Everyone was nodding.

"Men, there is no other option. No other option," I said. "Bless you and thank you for letting me walk with winners. Great job, men. Great job."

The memory of the guys chanting, "Juiiiiiiiiice!" after that speech still gives me goose bumps today.

The following Sunday, John asked me to serve as the team's honorary captain in the AFC Championship Game. I hadn't been feeling very well that week, but there was no way I was going to miss the opportunity to watch the guys battle the Steelers in Pittsburgh with a trip to the Super Bowl on the line.

In the days leading up to the big showdown with our division rivals, the players wore shirts with the words, WHAT'S OUR NAME? printed on the front. John shared the story of Muhammad Ali's classic 1967 fight with Ernie Terrell. When Terrell continually referred to Ali as Cassius Clay in the prefight buildup, Ali took note. During the fight, Ali asked Terrell, "What's my name?" over and over again as he pummeled him. Ali beat Terrell and won the WBA heavyweight belt in a fifteen-round slugfest that night.

Pittsburgh had our number that season, having beaten us twice already, and we were big underdogs as the six seed in the AFC. John fired up the guys with the story of Ali, and a series of press clippings from what the Steelers had been saying all week. "What's Our Name?" became our rallying cry.

Unfortunately, we lost the game 23–14, and the Steelers won the Super Bowl over Kurt Warner's Arizona Cardinals two weeks later.

It'd be the first of many consecutive postseason runs that'd end in disappointment. The locker room was devastated after the loss, our third to the Steelers that season, but hopeful that we'd get back at it the next year.

John addressed the team with optimism, and Ray Lewis assured everyone that this was just the beginning. That spirit of positivity is something I love about the Ravens. From top to bottom, there's an unspoken agreement across the organization that there's simply no time to dwell on the negative.

24.

MAKING A DIFFERENCE

Never lose sight of the fact that the most important yardstick of your success will be how you treat other people—your family, friends, and coworkers, and even strangers you meet along the way.

—Barbara Bush

THE year 2008 was a special one for Chanda and me for more reasons than just football. Though my health had taken a turn for the worse, I was finally making my voice heard in the ALS community. With the help of our dear friends Bonnie Downing and Mike Gathagan, we founded the Brigance Brigade, an organization built to equip, encourage, and empower people living with ALS.

Chanda and I had a mission in mind when we started the Brigade. We wanted to improve the quality of life for ALS patients and their families by doing whatever we could to help provide necessary equipment, resource guidance, and support services. We were fortunate enough to have the medical care and resources we needed to face the disease head-on. Now we needed to do everything in our power to help *others* do the same.

Luke 12:48 says, "From everyone who has been given much, much will be demanded; and from the one who has been entrusted with much, much more will be asked."

We'd live by those words.

In the spring, I was chosen as the ambassador and chairman for the Robert Packard Center's annual run to raise money for ALS. I got a chance to meet hundreds of other people who were affected by the disease, and the event generated close to a hundred fifty thousand dollars for research. A group of my old Rice Owl teammates, led by Donald Bowers, raised funds for the Brigade down in Texas. Seeing all my PALS—short for "people with ALS"—and the overwhelming support that we received that afternoon had a powerful effect and led to an epiphany of sorts. I realized that everything I'd gone through in life had prepared me for the chance to further the cause of ALS research.

Bonnie and Mike helped manage the day-to-day operations of the Brigance Brigade, but every week, Chanda and I would receive incredible notes and messages from PALS in the greater Baltimore area. They'd say that our commitment to each other and God, as well as our dedication to tackling the disease head-on, inspired them in *their* respective bouts with the disease. It wasn't just those battling ALS, either. We'd hear from hundreds of people, both within and outside of the ALS community, who were impacted by our efforts. It was all so powerful. I'd made countless tackles and taken part in various cause-driven initiatives over the course of my football career, but nothing moved me quite like these people and their responses to our efforts. The Brigance Brigade, even in its infancy, was showing me a beautiful side of the human spirit that I hadn't fully seen before.

I was never one for the media spotlight as a player, but when Kevin Byrne, the Ravens' director of communications, asked whether I wanted to partake in a few interviews that season, I didn't turn them down. The NFL Network sent a production team and filmed a feature on my bout with ALS. A national sports reporter named Jim Corbett interviewed me for *USA Today*. Every question they asked, I answered with honesty.

When Mr. Corbett questioned whether or not I was ever afraid, I answered from the heart:

"Was there fear? Yes. But how could I not accept the challenge I've been blessed with? I have no fear of death because of my relationship with Jesus. I know no matter how this comes out, I'm going to win. I'm fully expecting to be healed. Every day I walk this earth, I expect the next morning this may be the day that I'm healed; this may be the day of a new breakthrough. Even if that doesn't happen, I'm not afraid, because I know I will live again."

I did both interviews and assumed a few people would watch and read them. But, in the weeks after both pieces ran, I received hundreds of e-mails and letters from individuals impacted by my words. I heard from families battling ALS from states all over the country, thanking me for my courage and the inspiration I provided them. I got one e-mail from a man in England. He wrote to tell me how much the NFL Network piece helped him. He had lost his fifteen-year-old daughter earlier that year and he didn't know how he was going to live the rest of his life without her. After seeing the feature and how I'd chosen to live my life in spite of ALS with the help of Jesus, he was encouraged to go on.

This was *it*. ALS provided me with an opportunity to really make a difference. Through my struggle and our work with the Brigance Brigade, Chanda and I discovered that we could truly change lives.

This was my true calling.

25.

KEEP FIGHTING

Success is not final; failure is not fatal: it is the courage
to continue that counts.

—Winston Churchill

PRIOR to the start of the 2009 season, Coach Harbaugh asked
whether he could address me in front of the team during training camp. It'd been a long off-season in which I'd suffered many
more physical setbacks, and I was ready to smell the grass and
see the fresh paint of the hash marks once again. During the
dark days, the ones where I just didn't feel like myself, I'd think
of the guys running drills in the sticky August air and find the
motivation to keep fighting. After several difficult months without it, the normalcy of my football life was finally back.

John did something very unique that afternoon. "Hey, team,"
he said. "I want everyone to get close together." All eighty players in training camp and the coaching staff on-site formed a

tight circle around me. "Get tighter," John encouraged. "Okay, now I want you all to *touch* O.J. if you can. If you haven't met this man yet, introduce yourself. O. J. Brigance is the epitome of the Baltimore Ravens. This man, here, is what we're all about."

At that moment, all the players—from veterans like Ray Lewis and Todd Heap to undrafted free-agent tryouts chasing their dreams in training camp like I was so many years before—put their hands on my shoulders, my back, and my arms.

Ray Lewis kissed me square on the top of my head.

The team erupted in cheers and went out and had their best practice of the week. I wasn't a hundred percent sure I'd be able to make it out there that afternoon, but I found my strength through the presence of those men huddled around me.

I had a strong team huddled around me off the field, too. In addition to the fine doctors and nurses at the Robert Packard Center for ALS Research at Johns Hopkins Hospital, I was now making regular trips to Houston to meet with Dr. Stanley Appel and his team of awe-inspiring medical professionals, as well.

God led me to Dr. Appel in the most amazing of ways. While I was fighting my bout with ALS, Chanda's grandmother was also waging a tremendous battle of her own versus Alzheimer's Disease. Serving as the primary caretaker for her grandmother, in addition to me, Chanda was traveling back and forth between Baltimore and Houston to be by both our sides. Though I'm certain this period of her life took a tremendous emotional toll on Chanda, she never let either of us see her defeated or distraught. Somehow, she was there for both of us always, with no complaints or resentment. People say that I'm strong. I always tell them, "You haven't met my wife."

While in Houston one afternoon with her grandmother at St. Luke's Hospital, Chanda saw a sign out of the corner of her eye in a hallway. The letters ALS stood out.

She walked over and read about some of the groundbreaking work Dr. Stanley Appel was doing at the Methodist Neurological Institute. Intrigued, Chanda asked the woman watching over her grandmother whether there was any way Dr. Appel could meet with me.

She said she'd look into it.

Chanda called me from Houston that day, excited about the work Dr. Appel was doing, but curbed my expectations. "He's one of the top doctors in the world," she told me. "It'd be great to meet with him, but I'm not sure how likely it is."

Later that night, Chanda got a call from the woman at the hospital. "I spoke to Dr. Appel," she began. "He said he would be happy to meet with O.J. Can he be down here next week?"

God truly was watching over us.

We made travel arrangements and I was off to Houston for a trip to Methodist Hospital with Dr. Appel, another innovative leader in the field of ALS research. He and his team provided us with even more hope.

When I got to Dr. Appel's MDA ALS clinic, he greeted me with a smile and bright enthusiasm. He was wearing a bow tie, a lab coat, and leather cowboy boots. Dr. Appel was *not* your typical doctor.

"What a beautiful day it is!" he said as he entered the room.

The buzz in his clinic was palpable. This wasn't a place where patients went to moan and wither away. "We call it a cocktail party, without the booze!" Dr. Appel said with great charm.

There was action. Patients were energized, scooting around on their motorized carts, and joking back and forth with the therapists and social workers. "We call ALS the 'nice-guy disease,'" Dr. Appel explained. "No other population of patients—no other group of people with any disease I've come across—wants to give back to their community as much as ALS patients. The ALS patient is more about giving than taking."

He said that we were a special, select few. We were fighters. We were courageous. We were brave. "ALS patients are not like the rest of us. You, O.J., are *remarkable*."

Most important, though, Dr. Appel insisted that there was hope. "I promise you, I'm not going to retire until somebody finds a cure," he assured me. "How could I ever stop what I'm doing? Watching incredible men and women like you get up and fight every day? How could I possibly even *think* of quitting?"

Chanda and I fed off of his positive energy. "The more positive patients are, the better they do. That's a fact," he told us. "Other doctors tell me, 'Oh, that's an old wives' tale.' To that, I say, 'Nonsense! Look at the data. I'll show you the evidence on the immune system.' Your attitude and approach absolutely matter. The immune system gets stronger with positivity."

Speaking with Dr. Appel, I found it hard *not* to feel optimistic about my future. He gave us as inspiring a pep talk as any coach or teammate I'd ever come across. Not only did he firmly believe that I could take ALS on head-to-head, but he was excited and ready to join me in the fight. "I'm with you, O.J.," he told me in his clinic that day. He then pointed to his staff and all the patients around us. "We're *all* with you."

One of the first things Dr. Appel did was make sure I utilized something known as bilevel positive airway pressure every night when I went to sleep. I'd been previously using a BiPAP respirator for fifteen to twenty minutes a day, but he insisted that I use it every night for at least eight hours. The BiPAP, he explained, would help open up my lungs and allow my diaphragm to work properly while I slept. By my wearing a simple mask to bed, my body would function better and I'd see significant results.

When we first met with him, my speech was very slurred. By the second and third times, it was unintelligible. But Dr. Appel wasn't the least bit fazed. He insisted that *speaking* wasn't the be-all, end-all, and that as long as I could *communicate*, I'd be just fine.

He told me about a jazz musician who wrote sheet music using a chip in his glasses. He told me about a college football coach who still called in the plays while hooked to a respirator and in a motorized chair. He had a patient who had lost the use of his arms, legs, hands, and voice—but still typed forty words a minute by moving his big toe.

He was so inspired by all of their stories. "It's not about talking, O.J. It's about communicating!"

With technology improving at the pace it was, and with life expectancies increasing each and every year, Dr. Appel was encouraged not only by my battle with ALS, but with the state of the ALS community as a whole.

His goal wasn't to change the world in a day. He made it very clear to us that he wanted to do three things: improve quality of life, lengthen lives, and stop progression of the disease.

We left that initial meeting feeling like we'd been given a new lease on life. With Dr. Appel's incredibly positive outlook and the amazing work of his team in Houston, the doctors and nurses at the Packard Center in Baltimore, and God's will powering all of us, we knew we were in good hands.

We don't talk about it often, but Chanda and I both know she didn't just happen to see the letters ALS out of the corner of her eye in that hospital hallway by accident that afternoon. That happened for a reason.

It was the work of God.

CHANDA and I had long viewed the date September 29, 2009, as an important milestone in our lives. It was my fortieth birthday. Less than three years earlier, we were told there was a possibility I wouldn't make it to forty. Well, I made it, all right. And to celebrate the big 4-0, Chanda and our friends Mike and Bonnie threw me one heck of a birthday bash.

They called it "Two Rings for O.J.," and the outpouring of love from friends, family, and colleagues was truly humbling. The party was held at M&T Bank Stadium, and many of the individuals within the Ravens organization attended. From players to coaches to owner Art Modell, there was a sea of purple and black in the building that night. Earlier in the day, the guys on the team presented me with a cake and sang me "Happy Birthday" in the cafeteria. They sang it with a Stevie Wonder twist. Trust me, though he may tell you otherwise, Ed Reed *does not* have a voice like Stevie Wonder.

My parents made the trip from Houston, and several of my old CFL and college teammates came, too.

Chanda and our team of committed Brigance Brigade volunteers used the party for a greater purpose. We auctioned off a Cal Ripken Jr.–signed baseball bat and game-worn cleats from various Ravens. Someone donated Mötley Crüe concert tickets, and we auctioned those off, too. A woman bid twelve thousand dollars for an old Ravens jersey of mine. In all, the event raised close to eighty thousand dollars. All the proceeds went to the foundation and our quest to further advance our mission. It was one of my favorite nights of my life, an evening I'll never forget.

A few days after the party, Ray Rice knocked on my door and asked to speak with me. I loved Ray and told him that I was always available to talk. Though my voice was nearly gone, I was ready to chat about whatever, whenever.

He wanted to know more about ALS. He'd watched how the disease had ravaged my body, but noted that my mind was still there—fully intact, the same as it ever was. Ray had always been a curious guy, both introspective and cerebral, and he seemed utterly fascinated by my condition.

A few days after our initial conversation, Ray again dropped by my office. He asked whether I'd be willing to meet his mother, Janet. He said that he'd been telling her a lot about me and he thought we should be introduced.

When Ray's mom came by the facility, she saw me and took an immediate step backward. "I've seen this before," she said to her son in a whisper just loud enough for me to hear. "I've seen this before."

Janet's mother, Leona, Ray's grandmother, had recently passed away. She had ALS.

I greeted Janet with a nod and she told me that her mother's body and voice both went quickly, and in less than a year she passed. Ray wanted his mother to meet me in person and see what I was doing *despite* the disease. "Mom," he explained, "O.J.'s the greatest competitor I've ever met. He's our greatest inspiration."

Janet embraced me, clutching my shoulders as she began to cry. Her life was forever changed by ALS, too. The disease took her mother long before she was prepared to lose her. Sitting in the facility with me that day, Ray and his mom pledged their support to the Brigance Brigade and offered to help in any way possible. I assured them that Leona's fight with ALS was not a defeat. She's watching over us. She's cheering us on as we all fight today.

WE went 9–7 and qualified for our second straight trip to the postseason in 2009. In the wild-card round, we traveled to New England to play the 10–6 Patriots. On our first offensive play of the game, Joe handed the ball off to Ray and he went eighty-three yards for a touchdown. From there, the team never looked back, blowing the heavily favored Patriots out 33–14 in front of a stunned Gillette Stadium crowd.

Six days later, we didn't fare quite as well. Peyton Manning and the Colts got the best of us in a 20–3 Saturday-night loss in Indianapolis. After a string of solid performances, Joe didn't have his best game, tossing two interceptions in the loss. Though he'd taken the team to at least the second round of the play-offs in his first two years in the league, the critics started to come out in droves. There were questions as to whether Joe Flacco would ever be able to "win the big one."

Trust me, nobody within our organization ever had any doubts about Joe Cool's ability in big games.

26.

DON'T QUIT

It always seems impossible until it's done.

—Nelson Mandela

EARLIER in the year, I was invited back to my alma mater for an event at Rice Stadium called the Celebration of Courage. More than two hundred people turned out, and I got to catch up with several familiar faces. Many of the guys I played with at Rice from 1987–1991 made the trip to Houston, and we had the opportunity to share some fond memories over sweet tea and barbecue. Coach Goldsmith came, and the two of us reminisced about some of our wins—the big ones over Arkansas and SMU—and the losses. There were *a lot* of those. "Too many to probably go through," he said with a big, hearty laugh.

I laughed like I hadn't laughed in years that night.

As part of the event, we launched an award and scholarship that'd be given out to a worthy and courageous Rice student athlete annually each spring. I was honored and humbled to see it called the Brigance Courage Award. Donald Bowers, my old teammate on the Owls defense, helped get the ball rolling on the idea. Chanda and I attended the ceremony and relished the love and support of my old school and hometown. I wore the Rice uniform with pride for four seasons, and I never stopped being proud of being an Owl.

Now the school was sharing its pride in me.

The first recipient of the Brigance Courage Award was a young linebacker named Brian Raines. A Butkus Award candidate in 2007, Brian suffered a major knee injury at the start of his senior season. He fought back to return to the field, only to break both bones in his left forearm on the first series of his first game back in the lineup. Brian underwent surgery to have a pair of metal plates and twelve screws inserted into his arm, and somehow made it back into the starting lineup for the big rivalry game against Houston. Naturally, he went out and had six tackles and the game-sealing interception in an Owls victory.

Where did Brian Raines go to high school?

He was a Willowridge Eagle, of course.

Young men and women like Brian inspire me. They give me hope that perseverance and fortitude are not fleeting qualities from past generations. Everyone's going to face setbacks—young and old—and that's unfortunately an unavoidable truth about life. It's how you *respond* to those setbacks that matters. In Brian's case, he got back on the field, played his heart out, and graduated with a degree in economics from Rice. I love Brian's story and was honored to see my name attached to his award.

The Brigance Courage Award has given me great joy over the past few years, as it not only keeps me connected to the school where I cut my teeth, but also keeps me tied to young, aspiring student athletes seeking to make the most of their lives. I am in awe of their unbridled ambition. The Brigance Courage

Award has served as further inspiration in my daily fight. Every spring, I can't wait to see who's going to be the next worthy recipient.

MY fight got considerably tougher in the early part of 2010. Though we'd known the day would eventually come, it was hard for Chanda and me to finally come to grips with the reality of my no longer being able to use my voice. In a matter of three years, my speech had gone from perfect—I was the host of a TV show for the Ravens in 2006—to slurred, to now fully gone.

There were several trips to the Hopkins hospital and various visits with their staff during this trying time. Chanda was my rock, as always. She echoed Dr. Appel's sentiments: "It's not about talking. It's about *communicating*."

The Hopkins staff introduced us to a high-tech machine called an augmentative communication device. With the machine, I could use my eyes to generate a computerized voice. My sight, still fully functioning, would now serve as my chief form of communication. I could use my eyes to trigger words from a computer database, and through the wonder of this highly nuanced device, I could string together phrases, sentences, and paragraphs. I'd eventually be able to program in all of my favorite sayings, or I could generate new ones. I could do it all by darting my eyes in all sorts of directions. The machine would take a while to grow accustomed to, but over time I'd be able to not only converse, but write e-mails, as well. There was a remote control for my television built in, as well as access to my DVR so I could record and view my favorite television shows.

We were introduced to the technology and amazed by the possibilities that it presented. Though it was difficult, Chanda and I tried our best to stay positive. I thought about what Dr. Appel said about positivity and the immune system and pumped myself up.

So, I wouldn't be able to use my voice ever again. How was I going to approach it? Another challenge. Another obstacle. This was nothing bigger than what I'd already been forced to overcome. When I stuttered as a kid, I found a way to get through it. I dug deep and relied on the support system around me. I discovered an inner strength and a desire to face adversity head-on.

When I first lost the ability to walk, I looked to Chanda, to God, and to the Mighty Men in purple and black, and unearthed the courage to adapt to the circumstances. Those first few months were difficult, but the guys helped make the transition easier.

Most of my time at work was now spent in the motorized chair, but it didn't mean I had to stop being the same competitor I once was. That fire within me actually led to a bit of mischief around the Ravens team facility.

"If I can't run fast anymore, I'm going to drive fast," I'd tell my nurses. I took great joy in zooming up and down the building's hallways like I was Jeff Gordon or Tony Stewart. The guys on the team would scream, "Slow down, O.J.!"

Then one day I came into work and saw something different about the building's hallways. There were O. J. BRIGANCE SPEED LIMIT signs all over the place!

Wilbert Montgomery, the team's running backs coach, put them up early one morning. They were hilarious. They all had different speeds—1.9 miles per hour for the long hallways, 1.2 miles per hour for the short ones, and 1.0 for the areas outside the cafeteria and the building's main entrance.

I took such great joy in Wilbert's joke. He must have spent hours drawing those signs up. The whole organization was aware of what he was doing and loved it, too. Everyone realized the gravity of my situation. But the love we have for one another—built over many years, battles, and countless shared experiences—allowed us to have some fun with it, too.

"You're like Mario Andretti on that thing, Juice," tight end Todd Heap used to tell me. I always responded by saying that I had places to go, things to do. They'd all just have to get out of my way.

Losing my ability to speak would be another challenge, but I was confident that I could handle it. God wouldn't have put me through it if I weren't capable.

Whenever I went to meet with my doctors during this period of my life, I remember looking around and thinking, *Man, I've got it good. I have family who loves me and an organization behind me. I get to do what I love each and every day.* Reminding myself of how fortunate I was and how good I had it was an integral part of facing every new challenge.

We're all dealing with our own adversity. But how we choose to deal with it is what matters. All we can ask is, "How can we make life better?" Even when things appear dire, it cannot always be about "Why?"

It has to be about "What *can* I do?"

I could have let losing the ability to use my voice defeat me, but that wouldn't do any good. Instead, I looked at it from a different perspective. If I had been stricken with ALS even ten years earlier, the augmentative communication technology wouldn't have been available. I was fortunate to have the machine. With it, I'd still be able to communicate and share my message with the world.

So I did what I'd done my entire life up until that point: I got to work. I set a goal to master the workings of the machine and persistently kept at it. If Dr. Appel's patients could still write music and call in football plays from the sideline, why couldn't I do whatever I put *my* mind to?

My eyes, of course, would serve me in more ways than merely triggering the machine. I'd blink twice for yes and once for no. I'd roll them when someone—usually Ray Lewis—said something silly or absurd. I'd close them when I needed a moment for deep thought or prayer. I opened them to start my day.

If my eyes were the engine behind my new form of communication, my smile would serve as the steering wheel.

ALS could rob me of my motor skills, my ability to breathe and eat on my own, and now, even my voice—but it couldn't take my smile. I knew the great power my smile had. I promised to follow Dr. Appel's lead and effuse positivity for the duration of my bout.

I had my eyes. I had my smile. I had God. And I had Chanda.

I said it after every trip to the doctor's office then, and I say it still to this day—I truly am blessed.

27.

WORLD CHANGERS

I am not concerned that you have fallen—I am concerned that you arise.

—Abraham Lincoln

IN May of 2010, the Brigance Brigade held our annual Fiesta 5K run in downtown Baltimore. Supporters came out in full force, raising close to two hundred and fifty thousand dollars on a beautiful, sun-soaked day. There were three special guests at the race, though, who made the afternoon a particularly memorable one.

I hadn't seen my sister, Myla, in quite some time and was encouraged by the news that she'd be attending the race. Yet when she first saw me that day, she was visibly shaken. She kept her distance for most of the afternoon, keeping her two young daughters, LaGae' and Mya, close to her side.

This crushed me. I love Myla and I love her two daughters.

I used to take LaGae' to get ice cream when she was little, and we'd draw in her coloring books all hours into the night. Now she didn't recognize her uncle O.J. Little Mya had grown into a beautiful young lady, but she, too, seemed scared of what I'd become. Throughout the race, I looked in the direction of Myla, LaGae', and Mya, hoping they'd see my smile and offer one back. Unfortunately, they couldn't get past the sight of my physical appearance.

Hours after the event, everyone came to our house for dinner. What was supposed to be a joyous occasion was somewhat bittersweet because of my sister's inability to simply see me as me.

This is one of the hardest parts of living with ALS. Though I may not look the same on the outside, I am still the very same person I've always been. I'm still fully capable of seeing, thinking, smelling, and hearing like I used to. I am as sharp as ever, and yet people—loved ones included—often struggle to see me as such. They view me differently, like a lesser version of my true self.

Through the augmentative communication device, I told Myla that I loved her and I was still the same protective big brother who gave her prospective suitors the stink-eye so many years before. She smiled and began to get more comfortable, but I could tell how jarring the image of me, so thin and now unable to speak, was for my little sister. I gave her the space she needed, but made my way over to her two daughters. Though they were also startled by my physical condition at first, I could see their eyes light up when I smiled at them. I knew they'd recognize my smile. That hadn't changed.

They're my mighty nieces! Both of them are so smart and talented. Mya was just learning Spanish at the time and kept saying certain words over and over. Her thirst for knowledge was insatiable—just five years old and already working on a second language. All she seemed to eat at the time were red apples.

So, that's what we practiced in Spanish.

Through the machine, I said the words, *"Manzanas rojas."*

Little Mya smiled and responded, *"Manzanas rojas."*

Then I repeated the words: *"Manzanas rojas."*

She said them back to me.

After one more back-and-forth, Mya finally threw her hands up in the air and exclaimed, "Uncle O.J., you take too long to answer!"

We all had a great laugh at that, including my little sister. As the day progressed, Myla and LaGae' began joking and teasing with me, too. Any apprehension or discomfort was gone by the end of the evening.

I was so happy LaGae', Mya, and Myla were able to leave Baltimore that weekend knowing that despite the motorized chair and the computerized voice, I was still the same Uncle O.J. they used to play with down in Houston. I was still the same "big bro."

AS I adjusted to the changes in my life, the team adjusted to the changes in theirs. After the play-off loss to the Colts in January, Ozzie and the rest of the front office spent much of the off-season focused on bringing in additional playmakers to the offense. Anquan Boldin, a talented wide receiver from the Arizona Cardinals, joined the team in a trade. We drafted two young tight ends, Dennis Pitta and Ed Dickson, as well.

As was now becoming an annual tradition, Coach Harbaugh asked whether I would address the team in training camp. This time, I typed my speech out using my eyes on the machine and had our offensive coordinator, Cam Cameron, read it to the guys.

WORLD CHANGERS

As always, thank you for the opportunity to speak into your lives during this pivotal time. I say pivotal because there is so much uncertainty surrounding the league and our personal lives as a whole. Will I make the team? Is this my last season? Can I come back from my adversity?

Many of you have witnessed firsthand my adversity as I have battled ALS. Each day presents a different obstacle to overcome. From its taking almost three hours to get ready in the morning until bedtime, my mind, body, and spirit are under attack.

However, I know there is a greater spirit calling me to press on.

The spirit of Jesus.

I refuse to lose hope in knowing with God all things are possible, including my healing. One of the greatest words in life is *possibility*, and one of the most feared words is *uncertainty*. If we knew our destiny, we could feel some sort of relief and control. Only God is sovereign to know all things, and I trust Him to work everything out for His good.

We have all been assembled within this organization with divine purpose in mind. What does that mean? None of us are here by accident; nor was whatever you have been through in vain.

Everything as a player, coach, and staff has brought you to this place called "now" for such a time as this. All of our trials have prepared us to be world changers. We can be world changers by using the God-given gift within us to impact the world around us. Many of us don't know how we made it to this point but for the grace of God. We cannot let His grace be in vain or miss our moment of divine destiny. Many have missed their moment because they allowed outside influences and conditions to cloud their vision of God's calling upon their lives to change the world.

What does this have to do with training camp? *Everything!*

When we take the field, know that a trial is coming to derail our purpose and steal our vision. The great thing about our team is that the sum of experiences of overcoming as a family will far outweigh any adversity that attacks us individually.

Trust and rely on one another. Bear one another's burdens. Training camp is a crucible for finding the right men. Men who will stay the course no matter what adversity may come their way. This is our opportunity!

Are you one of those men?

———

WE started the 2010 campaign with a 9–4 record and had a crucial game against Drew Brees and the defending Super Bowl champion Saints. New Orleans had won six straight games and was surging toward the play-offs. Though we were the home team in the contest, few "experts" outside of Baltimore thought we'd be able to keep up with their high-flying passing attack.

I watched from the press box as the Mighty Men went punch for punch with New Orleans. Joe threw a pair of beautiful touchdown passes, while Ray Rice ran for 153 yards and a score on thirty-one carries. New Orleans tied the game at twenty-four, but we leveled the final blow late in the fourth quarter. After two Billy Cundiff field goals, the game was ours. Final score: 30–24.

We were victorious. Ray addressed the team after the game, telling the guys, "We've been through so much. We've been through every up, every down, every peak, every valley. We knew these were the defending champs coming in here. We got it done."

In the locker room, Coach Harbaugh told the team, "That was a great team win. All right? That's what we've all had in our heads. It doesn't have to be perfect for sixty minutes, but everybody found a way to have everybody's back. That's the spiritual side of us."

He took a breath and added, "We know where it starts. It starts up there, runs right through O.J., and runs through the rest of the football team."

Harbs then presented the game ball to me. A big "Juiiiiiice" chant erupted and I flashed my smile. "You'll have a speech for us on Wednesday, right?" he asked.

I blinked twice.

The Cleveland Browns were up next. In the days leading up to the game, I e-mailed back and forth with John and he again asked whether I would address the team.

Our offensive guard Marshal Yanda says my words carry so much meaning because I've always used them wisely. With a big game looming and the play-offs on the horizon, I felt like this was one of those times I needed to speak up.

This particular speech I titled "The Chosen Generation." I spent several days working on it. Coach Harbaugh did me the honor of reading it to the team prior to the game:

THE CHOSEN GENERATION

I was once again humbled by this team and organization for awarding me with a game ball. I realize that many hours of preparation, sweat and sacrifice went into achieving the "cornerstone victory" against the Saints.

We set ourselves up to be true contenders for a championship run. I can't help but remember the devastation we all felt following our last defeat. What a total contrast of the emotional highs and lows of a season. If you recall our last conversation, we talked about adversity coming and trying to derail us from our destiny as "world changers."

Adversity can be a great teacher in life if we are willing to accept its teaching and learn from it. My physical limitations have forced me to examine my character, heart, and faith. What was real and what was fake became exposed by the light of truth.

Now, here we are with a 10–4 record and the opportunity to make a running start into the play-offs with two weeks remaining in the regular season. What have you learned about your character, heart, and faith?

Some of you have endured injury, mental anguish, and personal disagreement this year. The key to capitalizing on our moment lies in what we have learned in the hard times. God uses what the enemy meant to break us, to mold us and strengthen us to be more like Christ.

In the Bible, the Israelites were God's chosen people who were to enter God's promised land. However, a whole generation was lost because of lack of character, unclean hearts, and lack of faith. What should have been a short journey turned into a forty-year excursion because of disobedience. An entire generation lost out on God's best because they refused to learn from their many rebellious acts in the desert.

Each season is like a new generation coming into the NFL. Every year, the roster is different from the next, and only one team gets the title of world champion.

Only God knows what the final outcome of our season will be, but we have a duty as "world changers" to use our God-given abilities to honor our heavenly Father. The journey to the promised land continues Sunday against the Browns. We can't miss our opportunity for God's best. We have gone through so much to get to this point. Continue to care for one another and bear each other's burdens and we will be victorious in the end.

We beat the Browns 20–10 that Sunday and took care of the Bengals 13–7 in week seventeen.

We went 12–4 in the regular season, but finished in second place in the AFC North standings, right behind our familiar foes, the Pittsburgh Steelers. We had a feeling that no matter what we did in the postseason, we were going to have to go through Pittsburgh at one point or another. The team leaders like Ray, Matt Birk, Terrell Suggs, Haloti Ngata, Ed Reed, and Todd Heap really didn't want it any other way.

As we'd soon discover, though, there'd be more on our minds than football in the coming weeks.

The Ravens are a family. From ownership on down, we're more than just a group of men who clock in at a job every day. We are our brothers' keepers. With this team, we all have one another's backs.

I tell Coach Harbaugh this often. Our corporate marketing may say that we're a team, but we're really a *family*. And when one of our family members is hurting, we have an unbelievable ability to surround him and raise him up.

Tragedy struck our team at the end of the 2010 regular season. Ed Reed's twenty-nine-year-old younger brother, Brian, went missing. Ed told me that Brian was always a loving kid. He had a son whom he cherished and that was his reason for living.

The team rallied around Ed during this time, as I knew it would.

He closed my office door following practice one afternoon and we prayed together. I couldn't talk or physically wrap my arms around Ed that day, but I could shower my brother with love and compassion.

No words are needed when there's love like that.

In the wild-card round, we faced the AFC West champion Kansas City Chiefs in their building. Kansas City had been playing good football, but there was no way we were losing this one.

Just days after learning of his brother's disappearance, Ed Reed suited up and played in the game. He made four tackles, including a massive third-down takedown of Chiefs running back Dexter McCluster. We won 30–7.

After the game, Coach Harbaugh handed Ed the game ball. Ed was understandably emotional. "I know my brother, and he loved football," he began with tears in his eyes. "But he'd want to beat Pittsburgh!" He led the team in a riveting chant. "One-two-three—Baltimore!"

The win marked our third straight year with at least one play-off victory on the road. It also set up a colossal showdown with the Steelers in Pittsburgh the following Saturday afternoon. We'd been waiting all season for this one, and we jumped out to an early 21–7 lead on the road.

John spoke to the men at halftime and Ray fired up the

troops before heading back out for the third quarter. We had a fourteen-point lead and all the momentum.

But it wasn't our time.

In the second half, turnovers did us in, and Pittsburgh came storming back. With less than two minutes remaining and the game tied 24–24, Steelers quarterback Ben Roethlisberger connected with receiver Antonio Brown for a fifty-eight-yard play on third and long. Pittsburgh punched the ball in for a game-winning score seconds later.

Final score: Steelers 31, Ravens 24.

After the game, Hines Ward, the Steelers' longtime receiver, told reporters, "What better way to put the Ravens out of the tournament? They keep asking for us and we keep putting them out of the tournament! They're going to be ticked about this for a long time."

Hines Ward clearly didn't know what John Harbaugh's Baltimore Ravens were all about.

That's fine. Not everyone does.

As he'd done so many times in the past and would do again several more times in the future, Ray Lewis gathered the team in prayer and kept spirits high after the loss.

"That's the past, men. It's done. It's over," Ray said to the guys in the locker room. "Football's a game. There's always going to be a winner and there's always going to be a loser. That's just how it goes. So, we lost this one. That's going to happen. How are we going to respond? We can only look forward. We can only push on. This is all part of God's plan."

Ray often tells me that I help put things in perspective for him. He sees my daily battle with ALS and it encourages him to ignore whatever temporary physical pain he's going through and to continue on. "How could I complain about anything when I see what you're going through, Juice? How could I even dare to complain?" he often asks me.

But the way Ray Lewis looks at things—his ability to view a setback and see light and hope gleaming through—always amazes me. He refuses to dwell on the negative and believes God never makes mistakes.

In that dank, dark Heinz Field visitor's locker room that evening, Ray Lewis saw better days ahead. "It's all part of God's plan," he said with confidence.

His will to believe is something I marvel at every day.

28.

PRESS ON

The only way to do great work is to love what you do.
If you haven't found it yet, keep looking. Don't settle.
—Steve Jobs

ANOTHER off-season flew by and another birthday came and went. I was now forty-two years old and making more of an impact as an ambassador for the ALS community than I ever made as an NFL player. The Brigance Brigade was doing God's work and impacting the lives of thousands. With the money we helped raise, we were able to get the costly augmentative communication technology to fellow PALS who were unable to afford it on their own.

I had a conversation with one of these PALS face-to-face, both using our machines to speak. We were doing the incredible.

Chanda and I were *changing lives*. My greatest accomplishment has been taking this personal challenge of battling ALS and using it to impact the world around us.

Dr. Appel was right. I have "the nice-guy disease." Just about every ALS patient I come across is gracious, humble, and brave. They say I inspire them. They inspire me!

Life's adversities serve a dual purpose: to refine us personally and to give us experiential knowledge in serving others who may be walking the same journey. Our adversity is never just for us, but to bless others around us.

The work I do on behalf of the Brigance Brigade is more rewarding than any work I did as an Eagle, Owl, Lion, Stallion, Dolphin, Raven, Ram, or Patriot. As I told Coach Billick in 2007, I was blessed to have the *opportunity* of being diagnosed with ALS.

I'm confident I'm making the most out of the opportunity.

Coach Harbaugh and I communicated frequently throughout the 2011 season, often sending daily e-mails back and forth to each other. After a big comeback win over the Arizona Cardinals, I sent him a note about something I saw earlier in the season that moved me even more than the victory. On October 31, I wrote:

> Harbs,
>
> What a great win yesterday. It will do us good to know we can come back if we need to. It was a win from the heart. Our way may not be pretty all the time but we got it done. The play of the season, though, actually happened about three weeks ago against the Texans. It was 11:47 in the fourth quarter when one of the picture runners went up to the head coach in the heat of the game. The runner didn't have a binder, but a quick hug and kiss for Dad. Of all the

things going on in the stadium, I happened to catch that great moment. That was an awesome picture of priorities!

Love you,
O.J.

We started the year 5–2, with a Sunday-night trip back to Pittsburgh slated for week eight. Losses to the Steelers had haunted us the past three years. Whether it cost us home-field advantage or it eliminated us from the play-offs, dark defeats to the rival Steelers seemed to hover over the team.

Ray addressed the guys at the team hotel a few hours prior to the game. "The moment is here!" he exclaimed. "We have been here three years in a row and have let this team off the hook! Make sure something else isn't taking you away from this moment, men, because it's all we've got!"

He had the team hanging on his every word. "That's what you guys don't realize most of the time. We don't get this again. The clock runs too fast! That's why we have to savor these moments. Because they're right now! I couldn't understand that when I was twenty-four or twenty-five."

He inched closer to the team and nodded his head.

"And that's why God incarcerated me. So I could see how great my blessing He had for me was. I had to be in a jail cell to be in the position to step on a Super Bowl podium. I watch enough film to put myself in position to let my defense be the best defense in football. We're not letting this team get out of here this time. That's what we're here for—a W!"

And a "W" we got. The Mighty Men played their hearts out and beat the Steelers 23–20 that evening. Torrey Smith, the team's 2011 second-round draft pick, caught the game-winning touchdown in dramatic fashion over two defenders with less than thirty seconds on the clock. Joe played fabulously, quieting his critics, at least temporarily.

It was the second time we beat Pittsburgh that season. We went back into the same building where we had dropped two play-off games in the past three years, and we left as victors. A page was turned. We were ready for anything that came our way.

Two weeks later, we beat a tough Bengals team 31–24. The energy in the locker room after the victory was electric. I sat in my motorized chair, right in the middle of the guys, taking it all in.

Coach Harbaugh quieted the team down. "Listen up. It has to be a great mental week all week. You have to study, study, study so we're ready to play Thursday night." Harbs then turned to me. "O.J., do you have something for us?"

Through the machine, I recited a speech that I'd prepared during the game: "Men, you did something very significant today. Every man stepped up and got it done. It is only the beginning. Get ready for something great. One week at a time. Here we go. Stay humble and hungry!"

Four days later, we defeated a talented San Francisco 49ers team on Thanksgiving night. This one had special meaning, as it was the first time Coach Harbaugh went head-to-head against his brother, Jim, the 49ers' head coach.

They'd meet again in due time.

In the festive locker room after the game, I again offered my thoughts to the team: "Tonight, on the night of Thanksgiving, we took care of our family. You know this was for our head coach, but this was for each and every family member who helped us get here. Know that as we continue this journey, we are chasing destiny. Enjoy your families and be blessed."

For the first time since John took over the head coaching duties in 2008, we won the AFC North division title and earned a well-deserved first-round bye in the play-offs. I wrote the coaches an e-mail on January second:

> Happy New Year!
>
> I am so excited and encouraged by the way you have handled the ups and downs of the season, keeping your hands to the plow, regardless of the outcome. My current state may not allow me to verbally speak to you, but it has helped me to become very observant of those around me. Beyond the words and actions, to the heart and intentions. Thank you for your will, dedication, and sacrifice for this team and organization. Every lesson learned during the regular season was in preparation for now! Congratulations and hold on to the vision.
>
> Love,
> O. J.

John asked me whether I'd address the team before our divisional round play-off showdown with the Houston Texans. I thought long and hard about what messages I wanted to share with the team. I thought back to our 2000 championship squad and the road we traveled during that magical postseason run. I spent the week crafting my speech, carefully editing and fine-tuning until it was where I wanted it to be. When the guys returned from their week off, we all gathered in the auditorium.

Through the machine, I read them the following:

SET THE PACE
Passion. A strong and barely controllable emotion.

Accountable. Required or expected to justify actions or decisions; responsible.

Committed. Bound or obligated, as under pledge to a particular cause, action, or attitude.

Excellence. The quality of being outstanding or extremely good. The state, quality, or condition of excelling. Superiority.

Good morning, men. I hope you all enjoyed some much-needed and well-earned time off. You are the AFC North champions and the number two seed in the NFL play-offs. Congratulations!

When Coach asks me to address you guys, I am always honored and pray God's spirit will tell me what to say. While preparing to come to the facility last week, it became clear. "Ray Lew" spoke with you about positioning yourselves to be blessed. Now, you have your purpose set before you. The purpose is to become Super Bowl champions. I want to let you know that everyone who plays this game desires to be where you are sitting now, with the opportunity to win it all three games away. Of the four championship games I played in, we won two and lost two. Let me tell you, it is more fun when the confetti falls for you than against you! We received rings, money, and T-shirts, but the memory of greatest value was the journey and men I shared this common bond with, as we pursued excellence. Three of them are in this room: Harry Swayne, Ray Lewis, and Wade Harmon.

That was our time and moment in 2000. This is your time and moment in 2012 to walk into your purpose and destiny. I watched the wild-card play-offs this past weekend and saw men step up their games for the opportunity to be world champions. Home field was advantageous to the eventual winners. Now, the Texans have to come to our house!

The Baltimore Ravens have a different makeup and DNA that the rest of the NFL has yet to see. Leaders, it is time to set a PACE never seen before in the play-offs, and for everyone else to match the PACE we display.

You set the PACE for the play-offs by playing with Passion. That strong and barely controllable emotion. You must be Accountable to one another to fulfill your role on this team to the very best of your God-given ability. Be responsible for your preparation and play. There must be a personal Commitment by you over the next four weeks to be an expert at what you do. Lastly, there has to be a spirit of Excellence in all you do. Not because a coach is asking you to, but because it is what champions do!

Passion, Accountable, Committed, Excellence.

If you set the PACE over the next four weeks, gentlemen, you will be world champions and we will give God all the glory and honor for the journey.

Thank you for this opportunity to share with you, and let's go to work and pursue our purpose! Remember one of my favorite quotes: "What lies behind and what lies before us is no comparison to what lies within us."

———

FOUR minutes into our divisional-round play-off game versus the Texans, the first postseason game played in Baltimore since 2007, Sam Koch punted the ball deep into Houston territory. The ball bounced one time before their punt returner, a young man named Jacoby Jones, tried fielding the ball. Jones bobbled the pigskin and fumbled it away.

We scored a touchdown a few plays later.

I remember watching Jones, an opposing player, and wondering how he'd bounce back from his mistake. It was a setback that'd undoubtedly haunt him over the following off-season. How would he respond to adversity? I looked forward to someday finding out.

Joe threw two touchdown passes in the first quarter and we never looked back. In the fourth quarter, with the Texans trailing by just seven points, their quarterback T. J. Yates lofted a deep pass down the sideline intended for their All-Pro wide receiver, Andre Johnson.

In a flash, I saw number 20 in purple leap into the sky and intercept the pass. Ed Reed had sealed the victory! The team had set the PACE, and I couldn't have been any prouder of the effort.

The New England Patriots and another trip to the AFC Championship Game were up ahead.

We didn't fear any team in the league, and we especially didn't fear the Patriots. We'd beaten them in their building in the play-offs two years earlier, and Ray, Terrell "Sizzle" Suggs, Haloti, Ed, and the rest of the defense had no doubt they could handle Tom Brady and his teammates once again.

There was plenty of history between the two teams. Ed and Ray respected Brady and Bill Belichick. Likewise, Brady and Belichick have never been shy in effusing praise on Ed and Ray.

But their fans hated us.

As Ray would put it, "We don't use the word *hate*, but we darn sure don't like y'all, either."

The team set the PACE early, and after a third-quarter touchdown pass from Joe to Torrey, we led 17–16. Another field goal put us up 20–16 before the Patriots took a three-point lead on a Tom Brady fourth-quarter quarterback sneak.

We trailed 23–20 when we got the ball back with 1:44 left in the game. Joe Flacco went to work. In what might have been the best game I'd seen him play up until that point, Joe showed magnificent poise under pressure. He completed three passes to Anquan Boldin for forty-one yards, and the offense advanced the ball to the Patriots' thirteen-yard line. A touchdown would win the game and send us to the Super Bowl.

Joe dropped back to pass and threw a laser into receiver Lee Evans's hands in the back of the end zone. Touchdown!

Or so we thought.

At the last second, Sterling Moore, a Patriots defender, swatted the ball out of Lee's hands. Incomplete.

Two plays later, our kicker, Billy Cundiff, trotted onto the field to attempt the game-tying field goal from thirty-two yards out.

Billy had made clutch kicks for us all year long.

Unfortunately, he booted the ball wide left and missed the kick.

Game over. Final score: Patriots 23, Ravens 20.

The team was devastated. We had multiple chances at the end of the game and visions of a potential Super Bowl trip to Indianapolis. But it wasn't meant to be. For the fourth straight year, the Super Bowl dream ended before we reached the big game.

Another group of men might have crumbled or been torn apart by the circumstances. There could have been fingers pointed or teammates shunned. But the Baltimore Ravens are not just any other team.

I watched the guys enter the locker room with looks of despair that night. They'd given their best effort, and yet it just wasn't enough to escape New England with a win.

I was curious to see how the team would react to this latest setback. I'd struggled with dealing with each phase of my ALS bout, and often found the strength and courage of others as my motivation to keep battling. Anytime I had doubts, I looked to Chanda or to another PAL or to a Ravens player and found a reason to keep fighting. The Mighty Men had just lost in the postseason for the fourth straight time and did so in heartbreaking fashion. A Super Bowl berth was theirs—we could all taste it—but it turned out to be elusive. How would they react? Who would step up and serve as the model of strength?

I, of course, knew who that individual would be, and couldn't have been prouder of the words that flowed from his heart.

Ray took the lead, as he always did, immediately absolving Lee or Billy from any blame in the locker room. He got the team in a tight huddle and said the following:

> It ain't about one play. It ain't about nothing. This year, we did what we were supposed to do. We fought as a team. There will be one Super Bowl champ crowned at the end of the year. So the way we feel? Somebody's going to feel that way tomorrow and somebody is going to feel that way in a week. That's a fact. And the fact is, we have to come back and go to work to make sure we finish it next time.
>
> Joe, you played your tail off. You hear me, man? Don't ever drop your head. Don't ever drop your head after a loss, man. There's too much pain outside of this that people are going through. This right here makes us stronger. Let's understand who we are as a team. Let's under-

stand who we are as men. Let's make somebody smile when we walk out of here. We have the opportunity to keep going, men. Let's walk out of here as a team. Let's be who we are.

Ravens on three. 1-2-3 Ravens!

29.

RESILIENCY

We have so much life in us and around us. I believe
you should think and look for the positive. . . .

—Jean Watson

ON a Thursday morning the following May, I woke up to news
that Terrell Suggs, our team's star pass rusher for the past decade, had torn his Achilles tendon while working out in Arizona.
The reports were grim: "Suggs tears Achilles; likely out for the
entire 2012 season."

Our team was no stranger to adversity, but replacing "Sizzle" in the lineup would be a particularly difficult challenge.
The 2011 Defensive Player of the Year was arguably the most
important piece to our defensive puzzle the previous season.

Paul Kruger, one of Terrell's backups, would be asked to fill
in. "Next man up, right, Juice?" Harbs wrote to me in an e-mail
that week. Paul was a talented player and a good teammate. We'd

miss Sizzle's fire and athleticism, but we'd have to do our best to hold the fort down until he returned.

The Suggs injury aside, the off-season had a relatively up-beat feel to it. The bitter taste of the AFC Championship Game loss in New England wouldn't go away anytime soon, but the guys refused to dwell on the past.

Come summertime, I was ready for football.

Harbs asked me to prepare something for the team's June minicamp session. I was more than happy to spend a few weeks crafting my next message.

On the evening of June eleventh, I addressed the team in a speech I titled "Next Time":

NEXT TIME

Good Evening, Mighty Men,

I always consider it an honor and privilege to address you collectively in a team setting. January 25, 2012, was the last time we were all together. I remember watching you men come into the locker room one by one expressing disbelief that we had not achieved our ultimate goal of winning our second NFL championship. I must say that I was astounded myself and tried to think of the words to say that would encourage us all, but had nothing.

Then came the words from one of our Mighty Men! "God has never made a mistake. It isn't about one play or player. This year we did what we were supposed to; we fought as a team. The fact is we have to come back and go back to work to make sure we finish it 'next time.' This right here makes us stronger. Let's understand who we are as a team and as men!"

Ray, your words brought healing to a heart-breaking circumstance. Your words galvanized this team and brought perspective to what seemed like a hopeless situation. Thank you!

Mighty Men, here we are five months later, standing at the door of "next time." We have lost players and coaches who were in that locker room last January. We have also gained players and coaches capable, ready, and willing to be the next man up. The vision and goal remain etched in the heart of this organization and every man in this room—to win the NFL championship. We aren't deceived about the amount of work it will take to get back to where we were, but we have men who have been tried in the crucible and who know what it takes to get back to where we were.

Every player, humble yourselves and glean from the wisdom we are blessed to have in our coaching staff. Rookies, follow the guidance of the veterans seated in this auditorium and you will see your learning curve diminish greatly. The table is set and the opportunity lies before us to do something remarkable this season.

I would like to conclude by sharing a bit of my weekend with you. Last Saturday, I had the opportunity to visit the Martin Luther King Jr. memorial down in Washington, D.C.

It was a picture-perfect day—except I would choose the very day when the Girl Scouts of America were having their hundred-year anniversary "Rock the Mall" sing-along celebration with thousands of Girl Scouts from around the country. As we made our way through the sea of cookie peddlers and pushers, we made it to this amazing monument. There was an ascending gray granite wall that had fourteen quotes from Dr. King. However, there was one quote that echoed in my spirit, as if Dr. King were standing before me himself.

It read, "The ultimate measure of a man is not where he stands in moments of comfort and convenience, but where he stands in times of challenge and controversy."

Again, "The ultimate measure of a man is not where he stands in moments of comfort and convenience, but where he stands in times of challenge and controversy."

Men, you have already stood through times of challenge and controversy. Billy, Joe, and Cam, to name a few, you have withstood the fire and come forth as pure gold. We don't know what will try us in the quest to make the final roster, to win the division, and eventually to win the Super Bowl, but know that every challenge that we have faced up to this point and will face going forward is preparation for our promotion, both spiritually and physically.

Coach Harbaugh, thank you for this privilege, and thank you all for allowing me to speak into your lives.

This is our "next time"! Let's go to work!

After a strong training camp and preseason, the team started the 2012 campaign with a 1–1 record.

We were no strangers to our week three opponents, the

New England Patriots. In the days leading up to the game, the guys focused on looking toward Sunday and not thinking too much about the previous year's AFC Championship Game loss.

I came to work every day that week eager to see how the Mighty Men would respond to the challenge of another meeting with the Patriots. On the morning before that Friday's practice, Ray stopped to chat with me on the sideline: "For me, every time you're out here, Juice, you click me back in," he said.

"When I walk out here, I tell the guys, 'Don't complain about anything.' For you to be coming up on another birthday, I just think it's awesome, man. Your spirit is just awesome, Juice."

The team was in a good mental state on Saturday night when we headed to bed. But we were awoken by news of a horrible tragedy early Sunday morning. Torrey Smith's nineteen-year-old little brother, Tevin Chris Jones, was riding his motorcycle in northeast Virginia on Saturday night when he ran off the side of the roadway and struck a utility pole.

He was pronounced dead at the scene.

Torrey, alerted to the accident by a one a.m. phone call, was immediately taken to his family by members of the Ravens' front office and coaching staff.

Torrey was more than merely an older brother to Tevin. Growing up in Virginia, Torrey watched over his six younger siblings while his single mother attended school during the day and worked overtime hours at night. Tevin looked up to him as a father figure.

When Torrey went off to college at the University of Maryland, Tevin took over the paternal role in the household. He picked up his siblings from school; he cooked dinner. Torrey was so proud of the man Tevin was becoming. His love for him was well-known around the team. The tragedy shook the entire franchise to its very core.

Torrey Smith is a remarkable person. One of the most beloved members of our locker room, he was a rising star on the field and a beautiful man off of it. He came to Harry Swayne and me early on in his rookie campaign and asked how he could get involved in community service off the field. His smile could light up M&T Bank Stadium.

But now he was grieving.

He'd never experienced death in his life.

The team rallied around Torrey as I knew it would. I'd seen this before: With Danny Barrett, my best friend, in B.C. With Jermaine Lewis and Ed Reed in Baltimore. Teammates have a special way of lifting one another up in their darkest moments of despair. I had no doubt Torrey would feel the collective love of the Mighty Men when he needed them most.

Ed, who'd lost his younger brother, Brian, less than two years earlier, reached out to Torrey first. He suggested his young teammate listen to a song called "I Give Myself Away," by the great gospel singer William McDowell. Though Torrey had never heard the tune before, the lyrics spoke to him:

I give myself away
So You can use me

Late Sunday afternoon, Torrey arrived at the stadium and told Coach Harbaugh that he wanted to suit up for that evening's game. John asked him whether he was sure he wanted to play. Torrey insisted that he was.

We dedicated the game to Tevin, Ray led a prayer in the locker room, and we took the field with far more on our minds than football.

Torrey Smith, less than twenty-four hours after learning of his younger brother's death, caught six balls for 127 yards and scored two decisive touchdowns. We beat the Patriots 31–30.

In the locker room after the game, Coach Harbaugh presented young Torrey with the game ball. "I wanted to thank all of you for your support," Torrey said as he clutched it with two hands. "This is new territory for me."

Torrey began to cry. Most of the guys in the locker room did, too. The emotions of the day took ahold of the Mighty Men.

"This is new territory for me," he repeated.

"Take your time," urged Joe.

"You've got sixty brothers in here," said Brendon Ayanbadejo.

"A loss like this, man . . . " Torrey said. "And if it weren't for you all, I don't think I would be here today. It's tough, man. I appreciate all the support. And you all really made me feel better. You know it's going to make this fight a whole lot easier. I love all of you. Coaches, players, all of you—I love you."

The whole team answered with a collective, "I love you," right back at Torrey.

To see his strength and courage that night further proved that there's no such thing as "impossible." To play the way he did, after what he'd just endured, well, what *can't* be done after seeing that?

As the team filed into Torrey's brother's memorial service a few days later, the first song playing was William McDowell's "I Give Myself Away."

Torrey had sixty brothers around him that day. He'll have those men by his side for the rest of his life.

Like I always say, our marketing may say we're a team, but we really are a family.

30.

BIRTHDAY BOY

I would rather walk with a friend in the dark, than alone in the light.

—Helen Keller

I turned forty-three years old on September 29, 2012. To celebrate, John got all the guys together in the cafeteria after practice. He read a quick message I'd written up for the team:

"'Strength is made perfect in weakness. So much is said without words spoken.'

"Think about those words for a moment," John told the team. "Just think about that."

I looked around the room that day and was overwhelmed by the guys' collective love. From the younger players like Arthur Jones and Terrence Cody to the veteran Ravens like Bryant McKinnie and Marshal Yanda, the Mighty Men were more than merely my colleagues—they were family. When the guys kiss me on the head, I take note of it. It was something only Ed and Ray really did regularly in previous years, but now it was an act that the rest of the team was taking part in, as well.

It's an amazing thing to see NFL football players—men in every sense of the word—exhibit their love for their fellow man with such a gesture. Through their benevolence, their hugs, and now their kisses, I could feel the emotional connections they all individually had with me. None of these guys ever had to *say* anything. I knew. They knew. As it's written in Proverbs 27:17, "As iron sharpens iron, so one man sharpens another." They were there for me and I was there for them. We were making one another stronger every day.

Coach Harbaugh presented me with an awesome gift that afternoon: a Muhammad Ali "championship" boxing robe in Baltimore Ravens purple and black colors. All fifty-three players and the entire coaching staff signed it. John placed the robe across my shoulders, as Ed Reed stood up and asked to share a few words.

"First of all, I just want to say happy birthday to you, Juice. You've always been a big brother to me. You inspire a lot of men. Still to this day, you inspire all of us. Happy birthday. Keep fighting, brother."

Ray Lewis followed Ed.

"Happy birthday, happy birthday, happy birthday a million times," he said as he clutched my shoulder. "Me and this man here have been through everything together. We've been through battle together. We won a Super Bowl together. I tell him every day, to see what he's going through as a man, there is *no way* any-one in this building could ever complain. He is our living wit-ness—no matter what you're going through, there is joy in every morning."

Ray turned to me and looked me in the eyes.

"Every day, when I run out to practice and see you there on

the sideline, watching from afar, I make sure that I tell God, 'Do not let me complain.' There's something amazing you give me. There's something amazing you give all of us. Happy birthday, O.J. I love you, Juice."

I quickly typed a message into my machine.

"All right, Sugar," I said through the device.

The team erupted in laughter. Ray gave me a big kiss and shook his head with a smile. I then addressed the Mighty Men.

"Thank you all for blessing me and celebrating another birthday. I never really made a big deal about birthdays, but now I have experiential knowledge that every day is an opportunity to live, love, and to enjoy. Appreciate where you are and what you have been blessed to do. Relish every moment—both triumphs and challenges—because we are growing through them all. You all give me the perfect gift of your friendship and respect. I am grateful to you all."

The team got together and Ed Reed urged for the "Stevie Wonder version" of "Happy Birthday." Ray kicked it off and the whole team got involved. Sam Koch was singing like Stevie Wonder! I saw Torrey Smith in the front row, smiling and laughing, being surrounded by supportive teammates Ray Rice and Michael Oher, and I knew the moment couldn't have been more perfect. No one had to say or do anything. So much was said without words spoken.

I was forty-three years old and my life was truly just beginning.

31.

THE LONG ROAD

Winning means you're willing to go longer, work harder, and give more than anyone else.

—Vince Lombardi

I have four nurses who work with me every day. They operate in two-man shifts and are by my side roughly twelve hours a day apiece. Without these fine men, I couldn't report to work every morning. Without them, I couldn't feel the love and the warmth of the Baltimore Ravens franchise every day.

One of the nighttime nurses and one of the daytime nurses team up and wake me at five thirty a.m. They use a mechanical lift to get me out of bed and into the bathroom to start my day. There, the daytime nurse will assist me in washing my face, brushing my teeth, and combing my hair. He then helps me get dressed and assists me in tying my shoes. At this point, he usually feeds me my breakfast. He puts my meals into a feeding tube and I'm nourished intravenously. Once I'm finished with breakfast, the daytime nurse will get me into the van and I start to think about my agenda for the rest of the day.

We drive fifteen minutes to the Ravens facility, the daytime nurse helps get me out of the van, and I enter the doors of 1 Winning Drive. It takes me roughly three hours to get ready for work every morning, but I don't know what life would be like without it.

Every time I enter the building, I feel triumphant.

Ray Rice tells me that the noise of my respiratory machine soothes him. "I feel good! I know Juice is in the building," he says. John Harbaugh called the hum of the machine the sound track to our team's journey. I don't know about all of that, but I'm happy to provide whatever comfort or sound track the Mighty Men may need. I'm also there to keep them going. Throughout my bout with ALS, I've made a point to send messages to the different men and women within the organization if I felt they needed some inspiration. From my vantage point, whether it's on the practice field watching from the sideline or in the facility taking it all in from my office, I get to see it all. If there's anything I can do to help, I try to do it. Sometimes, that's a conversation behind closed doors. Other times, it's a simple two-line e-mail to wake them up with a smile. Through my struggle, I've learned just how important smiling can be.

THE 2012 Ravens had their share of setbacks.

In early October, we lost our top cornerback, Lardarius Webb, for the season with a torn ACL. I love "Webby," a smaller-school guy like myself who'd risen above expectations to become one of the elite cornerbacks in the league. I knew how far he'd come, and to be lost for an entire season must have hurt his soul. I sent him many e-mails throughout the following weeks, lifting him up with biblical passages and the assurance that it would all be okay. God wouldn't do this to him without good reason.

In the weeks that followed, we lost Jah Reid and linebacker Jameel McClain to injuries for the remainder of the year, too. But no injury stung the team more than the one suffered by our fearless leader.

A few days after a week six win over the Dallas Cowboys, Ray Lewis gathered the team in front of him after practice. He had torn his triceps in the victory and knew it was serious. Ray never missed games. Ray seldom missed snaps. But this injury was different.

He shared with the team that the injury was, indeed, quite severe and that the team doctors had just notified him that he'd be out for the remainder of the regular season.

The room went silent. The Baltimore Ravens without Ray Lewis leading the way? This was new territory for all of us.

"Next man up," I wrote in an e-mail to Harbs that afternoon. Ray's presence would be missed dearly on the field, but his presence around the facility and in the locker room would be missed even more. He went down to Florida, where he began rehabbing with great ferocity.

Without Ray in the building, I was curious to see who on the team would step up and be a leader. I wasn't surprised when Ray Rice—or Simba—came to the forefront. He began speaking up more and serving as a positive example for the younger guys in the locker room. He even *sounded* like Ray Lewis. His emergence during this period made me so incredibly proud. I remembered Ray when he was a young rookie in 2008, just hoping to prove his doubters wrong. Now he was in front of the team, giving the type of inspired speeches his big brother had done for years.

Though we eventually got Terrell Suggs back from injury, the team began to falter. A loss to Houston, then two straight losses to the rival Steelers and Redskins, had the fan base concerned. After the defeat in Washington, John made a decision that I know was incredibly difficult for him.

Fourteen weeks into the season, he fired his offensive coordinator and our dear friend, Cam Cameron. Cam had been with the team since 2008, and I know how close he and John are. I was saddened to see Cam go. We'd been through a lot together. Jim Caldwell took over play-calling duties, something Cam had been responsible for the past several seasons.

The following week, we lost 34–17 to Peyton Manning and the Denver Broncos in our building. It was Manning's ninth straight win over the Ravens.

Three consecutive losses. In John's five years of coaching the team and Joe's five years of being the team's starting quarterback, the Ravens had *never* lost three straight games. The critics came out in droves. Everywhere you read, the Ravens were being written off. I reminded Harbs of Bishop T. D. Jakes's line about doubters: "Don't view them as haters. View them as stimulators."

I was interested to see how the team would respond to this latest form of adversity. Naturally, John never wavered. Due to losses by the Bengals and Steelers two weeks earlier, the team actually clinched a play-off berth despite the recent string of defeats.

"We're going to the play-offs, gentlemen," he told the guys. "You can't worry about yesterday. Only tomorrow." He cited Romans 8:28: "We know that in all things God works for the good of those who love Him, who have been called according to His purpose."

We had the defending Super Bowl champion New York Giants coming to Baltimore that Sunday, just two days before Christmas. I reached out to John over e-mail and shared my thoughts:

Harbs,

Through it all, these men have leaned on one another and refused to give in. The family is being built through these trials. We wear a tribute patch for Mr. Modell on our collars corporately, while each man has his own personal patch on his heart that tests and inspires him to press forward despite the circumstance. There is a process we must all go through to be called mature, but we know that all things worked together for the good of those who love Him and have been called according to His purpose. I know our marketing is team, but these extreme circumstances build family! We are growing stronger by the day.

Love you,
O.J.

THE team went out and played their most complete game of the season that Sunday. Though he didn't suit up, Ray fired up the guys with a riveting pregame speech on the field, and "Sizzle" got the pass rush going early. Joe threw for 309 yards and two touchdowns—one to Torrey, one to Ray Rice—and the defense held the Giants to just 186 yards of offense. It was a dominant 33–14 win—the perfect Christmas gift for the Ravens fans.

We clinched the AFC North division title for the second straight season and looked toward the play-offs. Through all the adversity, we were now just four games away from hoisting the Lombardi Trophy.

32.

AMAZING THINGS

With the new day comes new strength and new thoughts.

—Eleanor Roosevelt

A few days before we took on the Indianapolis Colts in the wild-card round of the play-offs, Ray Lewis knocked on my door and asked whether he could take a seat in my office.

"Juice, I feel like it's time," he said. "I feel like after seventeen years, I'm ready for life's next chapter. God's telling me that it's time."

He then gathered the team together and told the guys that he wanted to share with them two pieces of news.

First, he wanted everyone to know that he'd be playing in Sunday's game, just two months after tearing his triceps. There was no way he'd miss the play-offs. We all knew he'd make it back.

Second, he shared with the team that he'd made a decision. He was going to retire at the end of the postseason.

I could tell that very few of the Ravens players around me were expecting this bit of information. Ray kept his decision quiet for weeks, but came to this conclusion while getting the opportunity to briefly step away from the game during his time rehabbing.

His announcement inspired the team to new heights. They had plenty to play for already, but getting Ray Lewis another Super Bowl ring in his final play-off run was something entirely different. It motivated all fifty-three players and the coaching staff to raise their respective games even more. Work harder. Be better teammates. Be better men. Every single person in the building knew that they'd have to be at their very best for the following month.

Ray dropped by my office once more later in the week. He told me that while he was rehabbing down in Florida, he often thought of the many summer days he saw me on the sideline watching the team practice. When the pain was too great or the mountain seemed too high, he "thought of Juice" and my daily struggle. "From the moment we met, you've always been my greatest motivation," Ray said.

He noted that the media would talk about "my arm, my arm, my arm." "Juice, your whole walk is why I am able to look at physical pain the way I look at it. Watching you, I know that no pain lasts always. My arm? I'd think about you. And then I'd think, 'My arm will be okay.' You kept me going, O.J."

He kissed me on my head as he always did, and I blinked twice back at him. We'd been through so much together. I wanted nothing more than to see my brother finish his career as a Super Bowl champion.

One morning before the Colts game, Coach Harbaugh and his offensive assistant coach, Craig Ver Steeg, stepped into my office and closed the door behind them. Harbs said Craig had something he wanted to share with me.

On the night after the Giants game, Craig had a vivid dream. In this dream, Craig saw five men—John, me, Ray Lewis, receiver Anquan Boldin, and himself—praying to God for a Super Bowl championship. And in this dream, as we prayed, all five of us laid our crowns on the ground, and gave up all control to our Lord and Savior. We gave everything to God and got out of the way. Total selflessness. He would steer us. Craig had a vision.

What Craig didn't know was that the morning of the Giants game, I sent an e-mail to John, discussing the NFL's version of the "Triple Crown"—the division, conference, and league championship trophies. I detailed the importance of the word *crown* and what it symbolizes.

Sitting in my office that day, Craig and John appeared changed. They saw a clear connection between Craig's dream and my e-mail. Harbs looked at me with a smile and said, "We want to follow Craig's vision, O.J."

It was perfect.

Before every great journey, God's chosen come together to lead us. That's the way He deals with His servants—through dreams. And we were all ready to listen.

Ray and Anquan were called in. Ray asked whether he could bring Li'l Ray in the room, too. Together, the six of us went into deep prayer. Each of us said something beautiful. None of it was about football. It was about love. It was about brotherhood. It was about survival.

Ray Rice didn't say anything, but he observed it all. I could tell how much he was moved by the experience. Everything said in that room was unselfish and pure. It was about the betterment of somebody else or the betterment of the world.

On Sunday morning before kickoff, our team chaplain, Reverend Rod Hairston, asked Ray whether he would lead the team in prayer all the way through the play-offs.

Craig's dream and vision were now being spread through the entire organization. Ray said, "If we're going to be bold enough to ask God for a Super Bowl, then we have to be so bold to agree that every time we pray, we'll put our crowns on the floor."

Before Reverend Hairston preached, the whole team put its faith on the floor.

The spiritual power in the building was incredible that morning. When man completely lets go and lets God lift him, it's truly a beautiful thing to witness. Collectively, we joined as one. He was carrying us.

We all felt it. From John to Craig to the guys taking the field, it was clear. Even without any words being spoken, we all knew—the 2012 Ravens were about to embark on a very special play-off run.

Ray did one last "squirrel dance" in front of the Baltimore crowd that day and the fans loved it. We won 24–9. Fifteen minutes after the final whistle, there were still fifty thousand people dressed in purple, black, and white in the stands, showering him with unbridled love.

In the locker room after the win, Coach Harbaugh addressed Ray in front of the team: "There aren't even words to describe how blessed and how fortunate and how incredibly wonderful this week has been. I want to thank the guys on your behalf for making it possible to go one more week. You're a great man and a great friend. Thanks for being there for us."

Ray took the game ball and said, "There is no Ravens without Art Modell. There is no Ravens without Ozzie Newsome. There is no Ravens without Steve Bisciotti. There is no Ravens without Dick Cass. This is an organization like no other organization in this world.

"We know this ain't our last stop," he emphasized, nodding his head. "We've got stuff to do next week, so let's come back and celebrate for less than twenty-four hours. Nothing else matters except the next game."

Then Ray turned to me. "One of the greatest people that I've ever met in my life is O. J. Brigance. Me and this man, we hoisted something that this team is chasing right now. We once hoisted the Lombardi Trophy for this city. We held it. This man has taught me everything there is. Don't ever complain in life. Don't waste time in life, either."

I looked around the team and saw my Mighty Men all nodding their heads and looking back at me.

"He is the role model," Ray continued. "He is the example of what it means to be faced with crucial circumstances, and if you have the right mind-set, you can live through anything and do whatever you want to do. Ravens, this is just the beginning, men!"

The locker room gave its now signature "Juiiiiiiiiiiice!" chant, and I received kisses and hugs from just about everyone.

What a night. What a win for Ray.

Prior to the Colts game, ESPN aired a feature about my life, titled "Heart of the Ravens." I got to narrate the piece through my augmentative speaking device, something I'd never done before. They showed a series of highlights from when I was a player, and the guys on the team spoke about how much I influenced them. It was a very special segment to watch, but I was moved most by the response.

At the end, ESPN's Suzy Kolber and my old teammate Trent Dilfer mentioned the Brigance Brigade and the fine work we were doing. In the days that followed, the e-mails, the letters, and the support from all over the country came flowing in. Chanda and I were truly blessed. When we launched the Brigade in 2008, we wanted to make a difference and change lives.

Neither of us had any idea just how much of an impact we could make.

Five years later, the Brigance Brigade was not only going strong, but was serving as a leading instrument in aiding thousands of individuals affected by the disease. We raised nearly one million dollars for research, but we also met so many incredible PALS through our efforts with the organization. Now even more people were reaching out to us and offering their support. We were being introduced to hundreds of PALS we'd never met, who'd further inspire us in our fight.

Regardless of what we go through in life, there's always purpose wrapped within the pain. It all boils down to this: Every triumph and tragedy in my life has served as preparation to stand firm in this moment. To take what many perceive as an unbearable circumstance and be able to impact the lives of others.

That's what living is all about.

The team spent the following week preparing for a trip to Denver, where they'd face Peyton Manning and the red-hot Broncos the following Saturday night. I did not plan on making the trip for the AFC divisional-round game, but I wanted to share my thoughts with the team before they took the field.

I sent John a speech that I'd been working on and requested that he read it to the guys. On the Saturday night before the Denver game, he did me that honor, sharing the following with the team:

> My Mighty Men,
>
> As we await our destiny tomorrow, I wanted to share something with you that I have never spoken of—my time in Johns Hopkins back in 2009. I could no longer breathe on my own and was admitted to the ICU. I had to be trached and

have three tubes inserted into my lungs to drain the fluid because I had a collapsed lung. I was physically weak, as some of you might recall, and very thin, weighing only 130 pounds.

Not too long after my admission, another patient was admitted next door to me.

As I listened to his family and the doctors, I overheard them say that he was "DNR," Do Not Resuscitate. Basically, they were going to let the gentleman expire. If any of you have ever been in an ICU unit, you know it is extremely close quarters and you can hear one another's heart rate monitors and alarms sounding. For a few days, I listened to his breathing become more and more labored and his heart rate monitor beep slower and slower, until finally I heard the long continuous beep, and he was gone.

I found question after question coming into my mind. Did he have the opportunity to fulfill his dreams and ambitions before his time expired? Then my thoughts turned introspective. Have I done all that God had called me to do with the life He blessed me with? Was I ready to fight or would I let my life and dreams expire? Would there be limitations? Sure! But was my God greater than any worldly limitations? You'd better believe it! I decided to fight harder than ever for my wife and family and others battling this tough adversary, ALS!

I would venture to say that no team in the NFL has endured more turmoil than we have this season, yet we are still in the hunt, men! Our resiliency has outlasted our adversity. Now, the team that the world will see tomorrow is not the same team they saw in week fifteen.

We are Mighty Men, forged from adversity, ready to claim the rightful crown envisioned for us. It is time to fight like never before for your brother to the left and right, your brother to the front and back of you! We have that stuff on the inside of us, that spirit, which allows us to shine brightest when circumstances are the darkest.

Many outside of this team have set an expiration date on the 2012 Baltimore Ravens! They think our journey ends tomorrow, but they will be greatly surprised, because we never let what we see with our physical eyes deter our vision! Our expiration date is February 3, 2013!

To every coach in this room, thank you for your selfless sacrifice to pour your wisdom into these men on and off the field! Tomorrow's victory is for you. Have a great night's rest, men, because tomorrow we *fight*!

O. J.

———

THE Broncos were favored by more than ten points and hadn't lost a game in their last eleven contests. The odds seemed stacked against us, but I had no doubt that the Mighty Men could get the job done.

It wasn't looking very good with thirty seconds remaining in regulation.

Denver led 35–28, and Joe faced a crucial third and three on our own thirty-yard line. We had no time-outs left, and the Broncos were in a prevent defense. The offense needed more than a first down, here. They needed a touchdown.

Joe went back to pass and threw a long ball along the right side of the field. Denver had two defenders on the play, but I saw a man in white and purple bring the ball down. Jacoby Jones, the same young man who had fumbled the punt against us in the play-offs the previous year when he was a member of the Houston Texans, had caught the deep heave from Joe. I flashed a smile from ear to ear as I watched Jacoby, a Ravens free agent signing in March, take the pass and go in for a game-tying touchdown. Redemption!

It was incredible: 35–35. Tie game.

We were alive. In the overtime session, on a third and thirteen from our own three-yard line, Joe threw a perfect seam pass to tight end Dennis Pitta for twenty-four yards and a first down.

A few drives later, Justin Tucker, our undrafted rookie kicker, booted a field goal from forty-seven yards out right through the uprights.

Final score: Ravens 38, Broncos 35, in double overtime.

Ray spoke from the heart after the game, one in which he recorded seventeen tackles. He referred to Isaiah 54:17, telling the CBS sideline reporter: "No weapon formed against us shall prosper. No weapon!"

Ray was referring to all the adversity the team had gone through over the past twelve months. Last year's AFC Championship Game loss. The passing of Art Modell. Sizzle's injury in May. Torrey's little brother Tevin's death. Ray's, Jameel's, Jah's, and Lardarius's injuries. Coach Cameron's firing. The three-game losing streak.

The Mighty Men had faced adversity every step along the way and had taken it on as one. They'd taken on every challenge as a *team*. Their ability to respond to every setback and fight the next day was inspiring. Their focus and resiliency inspired *me*.

The next stop on the journey?

Another visit to New England, with a trip to the Super Bowl on the line.

33.

BACK TO BOSTON

We all have circumstances. Choose not to live in your
circumstance, but live in your vision!

—Chuck Pagano

A few days before the AFC Championship Game, John asked
me whether I'd once again serve as the team's honorary captain.
I was humbled by his request. The last time I served as honorary
captain was the AFC Championship loss to the Steelers in Pittsburgh back in 2009.

Just like that night four years earlier, the weather was cold
and dreary. Chanda and I made the seven-hour trip from Baltimore, and we both made sure to dress in many layers of clothing
on game day.

Prior to kickoff, there was an electric buzz in the stadium. It
warmed my heart to see the San Francisco 49ers, coached by Jim
Harbaugh, John's younger brother, had won the NFC Champi-

onship Game down in Atlanta earlier in the day. John was now one win away from facing his brother in the Super Bowl. He wasn't focused on any of that, though. He had only the Patriots on his mind.

My nurse and I made our way to midfield, flanked by the Ravens' captains by my side. Kevin Faulk and Matt Light, the Patriots' two honorary captains, both introduced themselves to me, and the official presented the coin. We won the toss, but chose to defer, kicking the ball off to the Patriots and giving our defense the first taste of the 2013 AFC Championship Game.

On their first drive, the D stopped Brady and company and set the tone early. Unlike their previous win over the Houston Texans in the divisional round, the Patriots weren't going to be able to throw the football with ease and run all over the Mighty Men. Prior to halftime, with the Patriots leading 10–7 and driving for another score, Ed corralled Brady on a crucial third-down stop. They booted through a field goal, extending the lead to 13–7. We'd squandered a few opportunities, but still found ourselves down just six points. It was hard not to feel very good about the first two quarters. I sat up in the Gillette Stadium press box with Chanda, with a contented grin on my face.

"What are you smiling about, O.J.? We're losing," she said with a look of great curiosity.

I knew things were going to go well in the second half. I'd watched the Mighty Men fight through adversity not just this season, but for the past five seasons. This wasn't a matter of "if" the Ravens were going to come back with a flourish in the second half; it was just a matter of "when." This was how it had to be. It *had* to be in New England, the site of last year's heartbreaking loss. We *had* to come from behind, with our backs against the wall. As I sat there in the press box during the halftime break, I couldn't help but smile, knowing what was about to unfold in the second half.

We punted on our first series of the second half, but got the ball back with ten minutes left to go in the third quarter. That was when Joe Flacco went to work. A twenty-two-yard pass to Dennis Pitta. A fifteen-yard pass to Ray Rice. A twelve-yard pass to Anquan Boldin. Another one to Pitta. Then a perfect pass to Pitta in the end zone.

Touchdown.

We led 14–13. Chanda squeezed my arm, trying not to clap or show too much excitement in the impartial Gillette Stadium press box. I flashed her a grin and blinked twice.

The Mighty Men didn't look back from there.

The offense scored touchdowns on their next two drives, with Joe standing tall in the pocket and hitting Anquan for both scores. The defense stepped it up to an entirely new level. The Patriots, an offensive juggernaut all season long, were silenced one possession after another. Punt. Punt. Fumble. Turnover on downs. Interception. Interception.

With 1:06 left to go, and the Ravens leading 28–13 over the Patriots in their building, Joe Flacco trotted back onto the field. He knelt the ball down twice. The clock read 00:00 and we were victorious.

The 2012 Baltimore Ravens were going to the Super Bowl.

In the most hostile of environments, Joe Flacco played flawlessly, putting to rest any doubts—forever—that he couldn't win "the big one." The only quarterback to ever win play-off games in his first five seasons, he'd now defeated Peyton Manning and Tom Brady in back-to-back weeks *on their home turf* en route to a trip to New Orleans for a shot at the Lombardi.

The team didn't run into the locker room right away. They took their sweet time on that Gillette Stadium field and savored every last second. Just a year earlier, they'd left New England without the Lamar Hunt Trophy, given annually to the AFC champions, in their hands. Now they wanted to relish their conquest.

I watched the team celebrate the victory with tremendous pride. My Mighty Men! Ed Reed, a ten-year veteran, was now headed to his first Super Bowl, and it was being played in his home state of Louisiana. Torrey Smith, just months after losing the most important man in his life, was going there, too. I looked at Harbs, who was clutching his wife, Ingrid, and his daughter, Alison, close to him, and marveled at his strength and conviction.

Last, I looked over at Craig Ver Steeg. He was shaking his head in amazement, somewhat removed from the rest of the guys. This was his *dream*. His vision. Craig saw this all playing out. I smiled at him and he nodded back at me with a grin.

It's hard *not* to smile when you witness something so powerful unfold before your very eyes.

The scene after the game was pure pandemonium. Uncle Earl was singing the lyrics to Eddie Money's "Two Tickets to Paradise" through the bowels of Gillette Stadium to no one in particular, as Sizzle was jubilantly screaming the word *Mufasa* in Ray's face, to the great delight of the rest of the team.

I awaited the Mighty Men in the locker room. A year earlier, I awaited them in the same spot, with great curiosity as to how they'd react to defeat. Twelve months later, they'd come full circle.

One by one, the players filed in, each Ravens player carrying with them his own personal journey. Jim Nantz, the CBS announcer, entered with the Lamar Hunt Trophy. It looked as glorious as it had when I'd hoisted it as a player back in January of 2001.

Mr. Nantz quieted the guys down, as Ray Lewis, Ray Rice, Sizzle, Anquan, Joe, Harbs, and Steve Bisciotti gathered around me. Brendon Ayanbadejo placed a BALTIMORE RAVENS AFC CHAMPIONS T-shirt over my shoulders as Mr. Nantz addressed the room.

"O. J. Brigance, the senior adviser to this team and a big part of the Ravens' success, is about to present a message that he's input into his computer. O.J. has been battling ALS since 2007. Through his computer, he is going to be presenting the Lamar Hunt Trophy to the Ravens. Here you go, O.J."

I blinked twice and recited the following: "Congratulations to the Baltimore Ravens. Your resiliency has outlasted your adversity. You are the AFC champions. You are my Mighty Men. With God, all things are possible."

As I finished my message, the team responded with, "Juiiiiiiice!"

Ed Reed walked the game ball over to me on the opposite side of the stage and placed it on my lap. It was a moment I'll never forget.

In John's postgame interview, he said, "Steve Bisciotti is the most determined guy. O. J. Brigance is the strongest man in the building. He sets the tone. I love you, O.J. And I can't say enough about these players. I *love* these players. I *love* this team."

And that's what it was. *Love.* What the men and women within the Ravens organization have for one another is what Ray Lewis refers to as a "godly love." When you feel *so* strongly for the people around you that every emotion is pure, untarnished, and mutually shared—it really is love. I looked around the room and realized that at that very moment, there was no place on Earth I'd rather be.

When Mr. Nantz asked Anquan Boldin about his two touchdown performances, "Q," one of the most spiritual men on the team, responded, "We have done a great job all year, but this locker room is filled with men of faith. All year, we believed no matter what the circumstances were, they couldn't shake our faith. All year, we've believed."

The Mighty Men—believers from the very start—were now Super Bowl bound.

In the days that followed, I got e-mails and phone calls from just about everyone in my circle of influence. Dr. Appel, Danny Barrett, my parents, countless Ravens fans, several PALS—everyone reached out to connect with me. They were all in my corner. They were all in *our* corner.

The Super Bowl awaited every last one of us.

Unfinished business.

34.

THE BIG EASY

Praise the bridge that carried you over.

—George Colman

THE media exposure of our unlikely play-off run presented unprecedented awareness for ALS and the Brigance Brigade. Interview requests were coming out of the woodwork, and Chanda and I were happy to do as many as we could.

One day during the 2011 season, I was introduced over e-mail to a man I'd long wanted to meet. Steve Gleason, a former New Orleans Saints special teams player, also had been diagnosed with ALS a few years back. Over the course of the next twelve months, Steve and I grew to be brothers-in-arms in the fight against ALS. Steve has the same positive outlook I have. He's a fighter, just like me.

Though we still hadn't met in person, Steve and I communicated often throughout the 2012 regular season and play-offs.

I'd encourage him with early morning e-mails and he'd keep me going with eloquently crafted messages of his own. After the Ravens beat the Patriots in the AFC Championship Game, Steve sent me a beautiful congratulatory note. He was excited for the team, sure. But he was also excited about all the additional ALS awareness he knew we could generate *together* in New Orleans when I got into town. We looked forward to creating the perfect media storm on the grandest of stages—Super Bowl week.

I did multiple interviews after the AFC Championship Game and started feeling extraordinarily tired. Because I used my eyes to type out all of my interview requests, I found them growing very weary. My vision was blurred and I was having difficulties seeing things from a distance. I just chalked it up to being tired after the long train ride from New England and all the typing I had been doing, but the pain wouldn't go away.

I spent much of the week after the AFC Championship Game in bed. The following Monday, I was sleeping so much that Chanda became concerned. I didn't think much of it, but she suggested we go to the emergency room and get things checked out. I was home, comfortable and relaxing on the sofa in my lounge clothes. I hardly felt like getting up, but my nurse got my shoes and we headed to Northwest Hospital to see what was going on.

I was very lethargic and could barely keep my eyes open. From what I remember, the emergency room was bustling with people coming in and out, poking and prodding me to figure out what was happening. A team of nurses drew blood, and Chanda and I awaited the results. I never liked hospitals when I was a child. Everybody who went into them never seemed to come out. I lost three of my grandparents to cancer when I was young. I remember visiting them and watching them shrivel up as the cancer ravaged their bodies.

I didn't see hospitals as a place of healing, but as a place where people went to die. As I grew older and matured in my faith, I learned that as long as Jesus was my Lord and Savior, death had no power over me. I came to tolerate hospitals after coming to this realization. ALS forced me to become more familiar with them than I would have ever wanted to.

We had been in the emergency room for a few hours when we finally got the results from the lab. My blood sugar had spiked to over three hundred and I was in danger of going into diabetic shock. My family had a long history of diabetes, but I never had any issues, because I always stayed so physically active.

The doctors sat me down and explained what had occurred. ALS caused a dramatic weight loss, forcing me to go from 220 pounds to 130 pounds in little more than a year. To combat this drastic change, I was put on a high-caloric diet that contained a lot of sugar. I gained most of my weight back, but because of the sedentary lifestyle I was now living, I faced a new health problem—diabetes.

First ALS. And now diabetes?

Really, Lord?

A new low.

Chanda and I took a moment to let the news register, then did what we'd done so many times before: We prayed. She did her best to lift my spirits.

"Nothing bigger than what you've already faced," she said with conviction and compassion.

Another health issue. Another obstacle. Another opportunity to overcome.

I was transferred by ambulance to Johns Hopkins that evening and admitted immediately. It seemed like homecoming week as I began to see many of the nurses and doctors from my previous stints in the hospital. I tried my best to never see them again, but here I was.

Hopkins had recently built a brand-new MICU, so the facilities were much nicer than they were during my last harrowing visit. As they rolled me from the elevator to my hospital room I noticed the number on the door: eleventh floor, room fifty-seven.

Fifty-seven!

It was the number I always wore as a player. It was the number I had on my back when I was a Willowridge Eagle in high school, a Rice Owl in college, and a Miami Dolphin and Baltimore Raven in the pros. The number held such significance in my life. It not only followed me for every step of my journey, but it set me apart from my peers.

I gazed at the room number. Fifty-seven. I didn't view it as a coincidence. It was God's way of assuring me that I'd be okay. It was God's way of letting me know that we'd make it through. He'd been there the entire time.

He'd be there for me now.

I refused to let this latest bit of bad news defeat me. It was Super Bowl week, and I held tight to the belief that I'd be in New Orleans with the team to witness the final leg of our journey. Also, we had several events set up with Team Gleason to promote ALS awareness. Being cooped up in a hospital bed for the big game simply wasn't an option.

The doctors worked frantically over the next few days to lower my blood sugar. They prescribed exorbitant amounts of insulin, and I was getting shots three times a day. I started to feel like a pincushion. This whole new regimen was overwhelming, because my body was responding slowly to the treatments. Our target date was Thursday. That was when the charter plane taking a group of Ravens officials down to New Orleans was set to depart Baltimore. If I could get my numbers down by Thursday, I'd be in the clear.

On Tuesday and Wednesday, there was minimal progress. It

wasn't looking good. I watched the Super Bowl coverage non-stop from my hospital bed to get at least *some* feeling of being there in person, but it wasn't doing the job.

Thursday—the day of truth—came.

We eagerly anticipated the daily lab results, hoping my blood sugar would decrease to a sufficient level that the doctors would allow me to travel. Dr. Todd Brown, head of the endocrinology department, broke the news to us that I couldn't leave. His words deflated me.

Friday's test results came and there was slight improvement, but my numbers still weren't down enough for me to be discharged. My hopes of making the trip to New Orleans began to dwindle. After all that we had gone through as a team, it was beginning to look like I would miss the most important game of all.

I realized being with the team at the Super Bowl was more important to me than I originally thought, because I started to tear up when I thought about not being alongside the guys.

As I sat there in my hospital bed with Chanda holding my hand tightly, I couldn't help but think of the Mighty Men. I wanted to make certain they weren't made aware of my physical state back in Baltimore.

They'd been through so much over the past twelve months and were now just one win away from making history. I feared that if they heard about the current state of my condition, they'd be distracted. There was enough on their minds already; they didn't need to be worrying about me.

Dr. Brown and his team still thought there was a chance they could release me Saturday morning if my numbers went down, and I clung to that hope.

I remained positive, thinking of Psalm 31:24: "Be strong and take heart, all you who hope in the Lord."

Chanda and I prayed together that Friday night. Prayer's

been such an important part of our fight. When things really get tough, I turn to God. He guides me. I wasn't finished battling just yet. Together, with God watching over us, Chanda and I were confident that our prayers would be answered.

I woke up the next morning feeling slightly better. We waited with bated breath in hope that Saturday would be the day. The lab results came in and Dr. Brown entered the room with a smile.

"O.J., your numbers went down significantly," he said. "My friend, you're good to go."

Do it, God!

The discharge papers came and we were on our way. Delighted by the great news, Chanda and I clutched each other tightly and praised God. At the very least, I wouldn't be watching Super Bowl XLVII from a hospital bed. As we took a moment to acknowledge how fortunate we were, Chanda got a call from someone within the Ravens organization.

"Really? Okay. Wow. Really?" Chanda said into the phone.

I looked on with curiosity as her eyes began to well with tears.

"Now? As in right now?"

Chanda hung up the phone and hustled over to me. She went into full-on head-coach mode.

"O.J., we need to get you up out of this bed and washed up. We're running home to get changed and packed, and then we're heading to the airport. We're going to New Orleans!"

As it turns out, Steve Bisciotti and Dick Cass had been in constant contact with Chanda and the folks at Hopkins throughout the week. They were both monitoring my health from afar. When the staff shared that I'd made a recovery, the team arranged for a private jet to scoop me up from Baltimore and fly me down to the Big Easy before Sunday's game. With the news came a message from John Harbaugh.

"If O.J.'s up for it, we'd love for him to address the team Sunday afternoon before the game."

It was one thirty p.m. The flight was taking off at three p.m. We had to hustle!

We raced home and packed all of our essentials. Chanda took care of the clothes, while the nurses grabbed all the necessary nursing equipment. Mike Hernandez, my respiratory therapist, packed all of the essential breathing mechanisms. We hopped into the van, and my dear friend Dennis Drake hit the gas pedal! We raced to the airport with New Orleans in our sights.

Though we were fifteen minutes late, the pilot greeted us with a giant smile when we arrived at the runway.

"Way to go, Juice!" he shouted as we boarded the plane. "Let's bring the Lombardi Trophy back to Baltimore!"

What a thrill. Chanda and I were amazed by the recent turn of events. We didn't ask, "How?" or "When?" but instead decided to just live in the moment. Sometimes it's best to not ask questions!

On the flight down, I thought about what I wanted to say to the team the next day. I'd envisioned an opportunity to speak to the guys while I was in the hospital, and crafted the pieces of a speech together in my mind. Though it may be surprising, I seem to have my clearest thoughts in my moments of greatest despair. The words came right to me that week.

We landed that evening and headed to the team hotel. It was the same hotel we stayed in for Super Bowl XXXVI when I was with the Rams. I prayed we would have much better results this time around.

We arrived around six p.m. on Saturday night. People were everywhere, and the madness of the Super Bowl had taken the entire city by storm. Ravens fans were packed in the hotel lobby, waiting to get a glimpse of anyone affiliated with the team. We were greeted by our team coordinator, John Cline, and made our way to the elevators. Almost instantly, people began to recognize us and started calling my name and cheering me on.

The next thing I knew, a lady jumped out in front of my wheelchair to get a picture with me. I accidentally rolled right over her foot.

That didn't stop her from getting the photograph. I flashed a quick smile and posed for the picture. "Thank you, O.J.!" she shouted. No problem!

We hustled into the elevator, finally making it to our room.

The evening meetings would start at eight p.m., so I quickly freshened up and prepared to head down to the ballroom, where everyone was gathered. When I had a chance to look at my arms, I noticed that I still had tape and glue all over me from the IV and heart monitors. It'd been a wild week, not like anything I had ever experienced in my life. Praise God, we made it.

The players, meanwhile, had no idea that I'd arrived in town.

They'd soon find out.

At eight ten p.m., the grand doors to the Hilton Riverside ballroom swung open and I made my entrance.

What a moment.

Within seconds, the team perked up and bellowed a spontaneous chant of, "Juiiiiiiice!"

"The final piece of the puzzle has arrived! The Juice is in the building!" shouted Ray.

I saw John's eyes well up. He'd later tell me that any nerves he had prior to Super Bowl XLVII were washed away when he heard the sounds of my respiratory machine enter the ballroom that evening. The rattle and hum of my breathing put him at ease. Every concern, every worry—whether it be about the game or life in general—was erased when I came into the room.

It was at this very moment that I knew it was all worth it. All the pain, all the frustration, and all the fear of the past week—there was something glorious waiting for me in New Orleans. Everything I'd endured over the past several years, it all seemed to suddenly make sense.

I sat at the back of the room, just taking in my surroundings. This was the same ballroom I'd sat in eleven years ago, when we faced the Patriots in Super Bowl XXXVI. As the meeting went on, however, I noticed my vision was blurry and I started to feel ill. I needed to lie down, but hung in there until the very end. I'd made it this far. There was no way I was going to give in to the pain now.

We usually finished our team meetings with a video montage set to music. That evening's film highlighted the play-off run that brought us to the Super Bowl. One image came up that confirmed the message that I would share with the team the next day.

It was a photograph from the locker room scene after the AFC Championship Game. The image captured the moment when Coach Harbaugh took the Lamar Hunt Trophy and set it on the floor in the middle of the Mighty Men. The entire team bowed in submission and reverence to the King. It took me back to Craig's vision of placing our crowns at the feet of the King. This confirmed what God had placed in my spirit to share with the team: "Raise the Crown."

Harbs greeted me after the team meeting, and I asked whether he still wanted me to share something with the guys prior to the game on Super Bowl Sunday. "Absolutely," he said with a big grin. "We don't plan on taking the field *until* you speak to us, O.J."

I returned to our hotel room for some much-needed rest. It was a hectic day, but we knew we were where we belonged—with the Mighty Men in New Orleans.

Once we shut off the lights, Chanda and I finally took a moment to reflect on the past twenty-four hours. Against all odds, we'd reached the Big Easy. Like the 2012 Baltimore Ravens before us, no obstacle could keep us from Super Bowl XLVII.

35.

GAME DAY

Breathe. Let go. And remind yourself that this very
moment is the only one you know you have for sure.
—Oprah Winfrey

I got up early the next morning to put the finishing touches
on my pregame speech. I was having difficulties with my computer, though, which frustrated me to no end. Now was not
the time for technical issues. I had a very small window to
deliver my message to the team, and I couldn't squander that
opportunity.

The afternoon meeting was starting at noon and I was up
against the clock. If my father taught me one thing in this life, it
was to never be late. Alas, at twelve p.m. on Super Bowl Sunday,
I still wasn't ready. Twelve ten flew by. I could sense John's blood
pressure rising, as I knew just how important sticking to a tight
schedule was on game day. Once the computer finally started

working properly, the nurses hustled to get me together and down to the ballroom.

At twelve twenty p.m., Harbs greeted me in the hallway. We made our way into the ballroom together, where the entire team was waiting.

Being late was inexcusable, but Harbs gave me a pass. "We'll let it slide, O.J.," he said with a smile. He then gave me a giant hug.

John and my nurse guided me to the front of the room. I looked into the crowd and saw the entire team—including the injured players, like Lardarius, who wouldn't be suiting up later on—and made eye contact with just about every last Ravens employee. I saw the team's management and ownership, from Steve Bisciotti to Dick Cass to Ozzie Newsome to Kevin Byrne, and marveled at the incredible quality of character gathered in the room before me.

The team was taking the field in less than five hours to complete their journey. I was humbled and blessed to be given the platform to address them.

At twelve thirty p.m. on Super Bowl Sunday, I read the following speech through my machine:

> Good morning, Mighty Men!
>
> Twenty-four hours ago, I was in a hospital bed watching TV coverage of you men being asked the same questions over and over. Forty-eight hours ago I was very heavyhearted, not because I would possibly miss the game today, but because I wouldn't be here to witness the last step of this phenomenal journey. Baltimore and most of the country is all abuzz with anticipation and excitement for today's game. They really don't know the price that you all have paid for this moment.

I was asked a week and a half ago during an interview the following question: "This team seems in many ways to be a team of destiny with the passing of Art Modell, Ray's retirement announcement, etc. Do you agree?"

My response was this: "I don't know with all the different events and challenges that we have had this season that we are a team of destiny, but I will say we are a team of vision. We have faith in a vision we have seen to be Super Bowl champions. Faith is defined as 'confidence in what we hope for and assurance about what we do not see.' Without faith, no great accomplishment is possible! I believe despite my diagnosis, I will walk again. This team believes no adverse circumstance will stop them from achieving their goal of being world champions in football and life! The outside world says seeing is believing, but men of faith say believing is seeing! Many have physical sight, but few have vision to see past their circumstance to their promise."

Over a month ago, Craig shared the vision God gave him about placing the crowns at His feet. The first time he mentioned it was after we defeated the Giants to capture our first crown, the AFC North Championship. He had no idea that the day before I'd sent Coach Harbaugh an e-mail stating, "We have a crown to win tomorrow."

A crown is defined by Webster's as a reward for victory or a mark of honor. I wanted to talk to you all this morning to remind you that we aren't playing for championships or titles, but for crowns. Ralph Waldo Emerson said, "It is one of the most beautiful compensations in life that no man can sincerely try to help another without helping himself." To achieve any remarkable feat, your purpose must be greater than yourself.

As I watched the video last night, the one image that stood out was the clip of the team praying with the Lamar Hunt Trophy in the center. AFC champions and crown number two at the feet of God Most High.

There are five characteristics that I have witnessed that make each of you men worthy of the third leg of the NFL's Triple Crown, Super Bowl XLVII!

CROWN

Courageous: Marked by mental or moral strength to venture, persevere, and withstand danger, fear, or difficulty.

Resilient: Characterized by an ability to recover from or adjust easily to misfortune or change.

Opportunistic: Taking advantage of opportunities as they arise!

World changers: Willing to use your God-given influence to make a positive difference in the world around you.

Nonconforming: Not willing to conform to the expectations of others, but to defy the odds in every circumstance. You are trailblazers!

Tonight, gentlemen, you have a crown awaiting you. I want you all to know that I love you and thank you for being my inspiration.

> Enjoy your moment tonight when God will
> be watching you display your gift.

I finished the speech and looked into the crowd. After a five-second pause, something amazing happened.

The entire team got up out of their chairs and responded with a standing ovation.

My speech had resonated in the men's spirits!

The opportunity to share some words with the Mighty Men on the most important day of their professional lives was worth every sacrifice it took to get to that point. It wasn't just about the Super Bowl, either.

It was about being there for the fulfillment of their destiny.

It was about being there for the completion of the journey.

36.

CHAMPIONS FOREVER

Faith: it does not make things easy; it makes them possible.

—Luke 1:37

WHEN it was time to head to the Superdome, Chanda, my nurses, and I all loaded into the van that the New Orleans chapter of the ALS Association kindly provided for us that weekend. We were parked in front of the hotel, waiting for the police escort to leave for the stadium, when all of a sudden a man walked up beside the van, opened the door, and climbed inside.

It was team owner Steve Bisciotti.

Surprised to see him, I smiled and greeted the man who'd been by my side for every step of the journey. He then kissed me on the forehead and asked, "Juice, are you ready?!"

I blinked twice and he exclaimed, "Okay, then! Let's go do it!"

He kissed me once more and promptly hopped out of the van. I was later told that he didn't want to head to the Superdome before getting a moment with me first. That was Steve Bisciotti in a nutshell: caring, loving, and *always* there for us.

His actions speak volumes of his compassion and integrity. Chanda and I truly respect him and his wife, Renee. They are such wonderful people. That moment with him, just a few hours before kickoff on Super Bowl Sunday, was as special to me as hoisting the Lombardi Trophy.

We arrived at the Superdome and I went straight to the field to meet up with my fellow PAL Steve Gleason. We had been exchanging e-mails over the course of the past twelve months, but still had yet to meet in person.

I was thrilled to finally greet my brother who has walked in my shoes. Steve has shown an incredible tenacity in his fight against this horrific disease. We immediately linked eyes and were drawn together like two magnets. We asked each other how we were feeling through our respective communication devices. How were our families doing? What was planned for the off-season? It was great to finally see Steve in the flesh! What a moment. Two PALS, out on the field before the Super Bowl, having a pleasant Sunday-afternoon chat.

Steve is doing some extraordinary work through his Team Gleason Foundation. That particular day, he invited two PALS as his guests to experience the Super Bowl in the building where he played his home games throughout his NFL career. Steve has that warrior spirit—that stuff on the inside that will forever link us as brothers brought together by adversity. He needed to get back to his guests and I needed to go watch the guys warm up, but we both took a moment to mentally capture the scene.

We exchanged foundation T-shirts as a sign of mutual support, and parted ways. Chanda put the Team Gleason T-shirt around my neck and I flashed her a smile. Meeting Steve Gleason was one of the true highlights of my Super Bowl XLVII experience. What an incredible soul.

THE game itself served as a microcosm of our entire 2012 season. The guys started off red-hot, jumping out to a 28–6 lead, only to almost let it completely slip away in the second half. An unexpected blackout and long delay threw us all for a loop. With the momentum gone and the rest of the football-viewing nation likely counting us out, they persevered. The Mighty Men found a way to hold on. The same resiliency that had carried them through the many adversities of the 2012 campaign kept them bonded together in the fourth quarter of Super Bowl XLVII.

Joe played magnificently, as he had throughout the play-offs, but with four minutes remaining in regulation, the 49ers had the ball, trailing 34–29. As I sat with Chanda, we watched Colin Kaepernick, the team's dazzling second-year quarterback, march his team downfield and into scoring position.

With just two minutes left in regulation, the 49ers had advanced the ball all the way to our five-yard line.

Though I probably should have been nervous, I couldn't help but smile once again. It all made perfect sense to me.

This was how it was going to have to be. In his last game as an NFL player, it was only fitting that Ray Lewis would have to lead the defense on one last goal-line stand.

On second and goal, Kaepernick threw a pass to receiver Michael Crabtree, but it was broken up by our cornerback Corey Graham. The 49ers called a time-out and I looked up and down our sideline. The Mighty Men didn't waver. There was no doubt, from anyone, that our D would get the job done. This was what it was all about.

Their offense, our defense, and the right to hoist the Lombardi Trophy on the line.

On third down, Kaepernick rolled out and threw a laser to

Crabtree. He appeared to have caught the ball initially, but cornerback Jimmy Smith jarred the ball loose. Incomplete.

Fourth and goal. A Super Bowl title hanging in the balance.

Kaepernick took the snap out of the shotgun and flung the ball into the end zone in the direction of Crabtree. There was one man covering the receiver—Ed Reed. As I watched Ed defend the play, I felt a giant wave of triumph come over the stadium. The pass was thrown too far. No flags on the play. Incomplete. Turnover on downs. Ravens' ball!

A few plays later, it was official: Ted Ginn Jr., the 49ers kick return specialist, was taken down on the final play of the game, and the clock hit 00:00.

The Mighty Men had done it! They'd brought the Lombardi Trophy back to Baltimore. My eyes darted around as fast as they could, trying to capture the reactions of the men dressed in white, purple, and black. They were victorious. They'd finished the job!

I thought back to the locker room scenes in Pittsburgh back in 2009 and in New England in 2012. I envisioned the countless summer days where the Mighty Men worked through the pain and worked through the heat with this very moment in mind. Now they were champions. Joe Flacco, Ray Rice, Anquan Boldin, Torrey Smith, Haloti Ngata, Matt Birk, Sam Koch—every last one of them was now on top of the football world.

I saw Ed Reed, that old soul from the seventies, hoist the Lombardi Trophy for the first time in his career. I watched him pass it on to Sizzle. Then I saw Ray Lewis, twelve years after clutching the trophy with me down in Tampa Bay, hold it close to his chest.

Forty-eight hours earlier, I hadn't been sure whether I was going to make it down to New Orleans. A few days before that, I didn't know whether I was going to make it at all. But God works in amazing ways.

I was there, all right, wearing a smile as wide as the world had ever seen, with confetti covering me from head to toe.

As I watched the Ravens celebrate at midfield, I thought of Emerson's quote "To achieve any remarkable feat, your purpose must be greater than yourself." There wasn't one man on this team who put himself before the greater collective goal. I am so blessed to have witnessed the entire journey—from start to finish—firsthand.

John was holding the hand of Alison, his fourteen-year-old daughter, and hugging his wife, Ingrid. No man deserved to enjoy the thrill of victory more than Coach Harbaugh. He lived his life the right way, both on the football field and off. We exchanged a look and he jogged over to me, full of joy. "Amazing, O.J., isn't it?"

Amazing, indeed.

As the team filed into the locker room to celebrate the win, I caught Chanda smiling at me.

I gave her a look as if to say, *What?*

She stood there, shaking her head in disbelief. Here we were again, champions—both in football and in life. My Queen B had been beside me every single step of the journey. From playing phone tag back in college to long road trips in Canada to being told I had only a few more years to live.

And here we were, in February of 2013, being showered in confetti once again.

Before Ray Lewis would give me several on the forehead in the next few minutes, Chanda gave me a kiss.

"I love you, O.J.," she said.

I loved her more than she'd ever know. With Chanda by my side, and with God watching over the two of us, I knew anything in this life was possible.

Anything at all.

ACKNOWLEDGMENTS

O. J. BRIGANCE

Even the darkness will not be dark to you;
The night will shine like the day,
For darkness is as light to you.
For you created my inmost being;
You knit me together in my mother's womb.
I praise you because I am fearfully and wonderfully
   made;
Your works are wonderful,
I know that full well.

—Psalm 139:12–14

THANK you, Jesus, for giving me vision when I couldn't see a way, for faith when my heart doubted, and Your favor to go places and do things I had never imagined. Thank You, Father.

Many people over the past couple of years have told me that

I should write a book about my life. My first thought was, *Who would read it?* Then I thought, *How could it be done without hands to write it?*

God once again showed me all things are possible with Him. During the many media requests leading up to Super Bowl XLVII, I was interviewed by a reporter from Fox Sports named Peter Schrager. Peter heard my spirit during our interview and wanted to write a book about my life. I had long wanted to write my story, but didn't know how I would get it done. Part of the apprehension was the painstaking effort to type letter by letter, word by word, using only my eyes.

Well, after numerous computer malfunctions, pages of typing being erased, and typing until I was cross-eyed, by God's grace—you have the book before you. There are numerous people who contributed to the writing of this book. Normally it would take a year or two to complete a project like this. We were able to submit our first draft within a few months! Do it, God!

I want to thank Peter Schrager for his zeal and vision to see this project through. You pulled the stories of my life together into an inspiring work that I am proud to have my name on. Thank you!

Ray Lewis, thank you for writing a remarkable foreword. I am blessed by your friendship.

Jennifer Schuster, thanks for your encouragement and for sharing your editorial gift on this project. Thanks to Scott Waxman, Joshua Kauffman, Carey Deeley, John Maroon, and Penguin Publishing for allowing my journey to be shared with the world. Blessings to you all!

Just as a tree has countless roots to sustain its life, I, too, have many people who have touched my life by feeding me with their love and support. My life has been marked by triumphs and trials, but through it all, the root of resiliency has sustained me to stand firm. I have been nourished by many family and friends. Thank you all from the bottom of my heart!

To my Queen B, Chanda: You astound me with your strength and commitment. God gave me the perfect mate in you. Thank you for loving me through it all.

To my parents: Thank you for never settling for mediocrity and for not allowing me to settle either. To my grandparents, aunts, uncles, and cousins: Thanks for always being there.

Myla, you are the best sister a brother could have ever asked for.

To my brothers Karl and Todd: Fellas, we went through it all together. Thanks for allowing me to be me. You all always had my back—right, wrong, or indifferent. I love you, men!

I want to thank my team of caregivers who help me live every day to its fullest! Lora Clawson, Bill Shields, Paul Morris, Edrissa Njie, Raymond Ebai, Robin Navarro, Michele Miller, Mike Hernandez, and Angela Lane: Thank you all for caring so that I can complete God's assignment for me.

To the Baltimore Ravens organization: You have been an unwavering source of encouragement and support. Steve and Renee Bisciotti, thank you for being so giving to us in every way. Dick Cass, Ozzie Newsome, Brian Billick, John Harbaugh, Jack Del Rio, Cam Cameron, Marvin Lewis, Rod Hairston, Harry Swayne, Darren Sanders, and Top Flight Security, and every employee past and present, thank you for imparting kindness and strength into my life.

I have been blessed to encounter many Mighty Men during my time in Baltimore. Thanks for touching my life, Orlando BoBo, Trent Dilfer, James Trapp, Peter Boulware, Jamie Sharper, Brad Jackson, Cornell Brown, Anthony Davis, Ed Reed, and my rookie classes as PDD.

My time in St. Louis with the Greatest Show on Turf stretched me. Lovie Smith, Mike Haluchek, Bobby April, Dana LeDuc, Aeneas Williams, Kurt Warner, Don Davis, Ernie Conwell, Tommy Polley, London Fletcher, I experienced the faith-fulness of God through you all. Thank you!

God showed me that all things were possible in Miami. Bob Ackles, Jimmy Johnson, George Hill, Mike Westhoff, John Gamble, Brad Roll, Jeremy Fedouruk, Ryan Vermilion, Kevin O'Neil, Joe Cimino, Charlie Thiele, Stu Weinstein, you helped my dream come true. Thanks for everything. To my linebackers and special teams crew, thanks for the great memories. Michael Stewart, Troy Vincent, Dwight Hollier, Larry Izzo, Zach Thomas, Anthony Harris, Jim Kitts, Rickey Brady, Qadry Is-mail, Bernie Parmalee, you men made me better. Thank you!

We became the only American team to become CFL Champions in Baltimore. Jim Speros, Jim Popp, Don Matthews, Mike Gathagan, Bonnie Downing, Marty Long, Don Hill, Bob Price, Tracy Ham, Elfrid Payton, Courtney Griffin, Chris Wright, Jearld Bayliss, Grant Carter—thanks to all of my Baltimore Stallion teammates for their commitment to excellence.

My professional career carried me across North America and allowed me to meet so many great people: Bill Quinter, Bob O'Billovich, Dave Ritchie, Gene Gaines, Jeff Reinbold, Roger Kelly, the Hewlett family, Danny Barrett, Zock Allen, Keith Powe, Doug Hocking, Stew Hill, and Chris Skinner from my time with the B.C. Lions.

Rice University, you gave me a chance when no one else would. For that I am eternally grateful. Donald Dobes, Jerry Berndt, Ron Chismar, Fred Goldsmith, Keith Irwin, Jeff Mad-den, Julie Griswold, Allen Eggert, thank you. To my many teammates, it was an honor to play with you: Donald Bowers, Everett Coleman, David Alston, Will and Donald Hollas, Eric Henley, Courtney Hall, Courtney Cravin, Richard Williams, the Latin Brothers, Alonzo Williams, Mike Hooks, Mike Ap-pelbaum, and the rest of Owl Nation.

Willowridge Eagle family, you taught me what it meant to

have "Class and Character." Many thanks to John Pearce, Richard Campbell, Travis Vaughn, Eddie Brister, and the many other coaches who believed in me over the years. To all my teammates who sweated it out with me under the hot Texas sun, thank you! Ed Glover, Candy Anderson, Virginia Lister, Audrey Williams, Paula Jay, thanks for challenging me every single day. Class of '87, thanks for your support!

PETER SCHRAGER

Working on *Strength of a Champion* has been the most rewarding experience of my professional career. On a personal level, it's changed me. Thank you, O.J. and Chanda, for opening up your lives, your beautiful home, and your incredible story to me. Your love, commitment, and passion for each other and your dreams serve as the model that we should all look to follow. You're both incredible people.

This book wouldn't have come together without the tireless work and selflessness of the Baltimore Ravens' public relations staff. Kevin Byrne and Chad Steele, thank you for quite literally handing me the "keys to the castle" and ensuring that this book came to life. Your love for O.J. and your commitment to this project helped add the rich color and details that his story deserves. Tom Valente, Pat Gleason, Megan McLaughlin, Dan Parsons—thank you for all the amazing work you do at 1 Winning Drive.

Marcus, Barbara, and Myla, the conversations weren't always easy, but you were always wonderful and gracious with your time. Special thanks to Coach Dobes, Coach Coleman, Donald Bowers, Mike Hooks, Larry Izzo, Mike Gathagan, Christine Kirkley, Zach Thomas, Jason LaCanfora, Eve Hemsley, John Maroon, Deb Poquette, Ashley Knight, Dr. Stanley Appel, Todd McQuietor, Karl Lewis, Qadry Ismail, and Danny Barrett. Jimmy Johnson, you gave me as much time as I needed, and shared some wonderful stories from the Dolphins years. Brian Billick, you were insightful and willing to jump on the phone with me whenever I had any questions for you to answer.

John Harbaugh and Ozzie Newsome—it all starts with the two of you. Thank you for making the time to speak with me during the busiest of off-seasons.

Ray Lewis, thank you for your cooperation and the beautifully written foreword. Best of luck in your new career behind the microphone.

Thank you, Joe Flacco, Art Jones, Ray Rice, Torrey Smith, Marshal Yanda, David Reed, Lardarius Webb, Terrell Suggs, Craig Ver Steeg, Brendon Ayanbadejo, and Sam Koch. You're all champions. Thank you so much for championing this project.

Nancy Gay, many thanks for assigning a profile on O.J. for FoxSports.com back in January. Thank you, Rick Jaffe, Jacob Ullman, John Entz, Scott Ackerson, Michael Hughes, Chris D'Amico, Stephen Miller, Alex Marvez, Todd Behrendt, Ross Jones, Devin Gordon, Phil Simms, James Brown, Cris Collinsworth, Jim Nantz, Mike Lombardi, Gareth Hughes, the whole *Inside the NFL* crew, Eric Gillin, Mike Tanenbaum, Dan Craparo, and Pete Radovich, for opening the doors to such an amazing opportunity.

Scott Waxman, your confidence in this project will never be forgotten. Thanks for all that you do. I'll speak to Mikey's middle school class anytime you need me to, as long as there's some decent pizza waiting for us at the end. Jennifer Schuster, few editors could have helped O.J. and me through this. Thank you for your guidance and dedication to *Strength of a Champion*. Ray

Garcia, I have much appreciation for the work that you do. Talia Platz, thanks to you, as well.

Mom, Dad, Justin, Sarah, David, and the Hotel Hirshfeld—thanks for being there always.

Erica, you're my compass and my inspiration. You're my everything.

ABOUT THE AUTHORS

O. J. Brigance is currently the senior adviser of player development for the Baltimore Ravens. He created the Brigance Brigade Foundation to raise awareness and funding for ALS research and patient services.

Peter Schrager is the senior national writer for FOXSports.com and the sports correspondent for FOX News Channel's *FOX Report Weekend*. He's the coauthor of Victor Cruz's *New York Times* best-selling memoir, *Out of the Blue*.